8459

PREPARATION TO CARE

610- 730698 RIC

Withdrawn 21/6/10 m

PREPARATION TO CARE

A Foundation NVQ text for Health Care Assistants

Edited by

Aileen Richardson

**Training and Education Centre,
Harrogate Health Care N.H.S. Trust, UK**

BAILLIÈRE TINDALL
London Philadelphia Toronto Sydney Tokyo

NVQ

Baillière Tindall   24–28 Oval Road
London NW1 7DX

The Curtis Center
Independence Square West
Philadelphia, PA 19106–3399, USA

Harcourt Brace & Company
55 Horner Avenue
Toronto, Ontario M8Z 4X6, Canada

Harcourt Brace & Company, Australia
30–52 Smidmore Street
Marrickville
NSW 2204, Australia

Harcourt Brace & Company, Japan
Ichibancho Central Building
22–1 Ichibancho
Chiyoda-ku, Tokyo 102, Japan

This book is printed on acid-free paper

A catalogue record for this book is available from the British Library

ISBN 0-7020-1793-0

Typeset by J&L Composition Ltd, Filey, North Yorkshire
Printed and bound in Great Britain by The Bath Press, Avon

Contents

Contributors

Pamela Bradley
Formerly Chief Nursing Officer for
Harrogate Health Authority,
North Yorkshire.

Damon Britton
Ward Manager
Roundhay Wing
St James University Hospital, Leeds.

Elizabeth Bulmer
Contractual Trainee Member of the
Institute of Transactional Analysis
Mental Health Unit
Harrogate Health Care N.H.S. Trust,
North Yorkshire.

Paul Evans
P2000 Course Tutor
Learning Disability Nursing
North Yorkshire College of Health
Studies.

Fiona Evard
Back Care and Lifting
Co-ordinator
Physiotherapist
Harrogate Health Care N.H.S. Trust,
North Yorkshire.

Clare Fitzgibbon
Macmillan Nurse Consultant,
North Yorkshire.

Joanna Fogden
Senior Occupational Therapist
Medical and Elderly Directorate
Harrogate Health Care N.H.S. Trust,
North Yorkshire.

Rozila Horton
Clinical Nurse Advisor – Infection
Control
Harrogate Health Care N.H.S. Trust,
North Yorkshire.

Stephanie Pye
Senior Lecturer in Nursing
Sheffield Hallam University, Sheffield

(Mrs) Aileen Richardson
Senior Training and Education Officer
Harrogate Health Care N.H.S. Trust,
North Yorkshire.

Gillian Senior
Librarian
North Yorkshire College of Health
Studies
Harrogate General Hospital,
North Yorkshire

David Tordoff
Training and Education Manager
Harrogate Health Care N.H.S. Trust,
North Yorkshire.

Angela Turner
Senior Nurse Manager Quality
Assurance
Harrogate Health Care N.H.S. Trust,
North Yorkshire.

(Mrs) Kathleen Wheatley
Senior Training and Education Officer
Harrogate Health Care N.H.S. Trust,
North Yorkshire.

Judith Wilson
Senior Training and Education Officer/
Nurse Teacher
Harrogate Health Care N.H.S. Trust,
North Yorkshire.

Anita Wood
Ward Manager
Medical and Elderly Directorate
Harrogate Health Care N.H.S. Trust,
North Yorkshire.

Peter Wood
HIV Training Officer
Tameside and Glossop Community
and Priority Services N.H.S. Trust,
Mossley, Ashton-upon-Lyne.

Acknowledgements

The idea for writing this book came from the enthusiasm, motivation and commitment to learning demonstrated by the Health Care Assistants, with whom I have had the pleasure to work. Unwittingly, the students themselves were the inspiration, but translating the idea into reality has only been possible through the expertise of Kathleen Wheatley.

I would like to thank each contributor not only for the provision of their expertise, but also for their patience and dedication to this project.

In addition, I wish to extend my gratitude to Jacqueline Curthoys for her unstinting support, to Betty Kershaw for her initial encouragement of the project, my family Gavin, Nicola and Steven and not least Jane and John Mallard.

Aileen Richardson
March 1995

How to use this book

This book has been designed to be as flexible and as supportive as possible. This is because all carers have a range of different experiences and skills and everyone learns in different ways.

The chapters in this book do not have to be looked at in a particular order. However, to help you decide what you do want to read, each Section begins with a short introduction explaining what chapters are included. Each Section in the book covers topics which can be linked to each other and even if you do not think a chapter is immediately relevant, you will find that it contains information relating to other chapters in that Section. Each chapter starts with a short introduction, as well as a list of NVQ units (see below), so you can see quickly whether the chapter contains the information you need. By the time you reach the end of the book, you will appreciate that no single chapter or section is entirely independent of the others.

We hope you will find the book useful as both:

- a reference source for specific information referring to a particular NVQ unit, and
- a textbook if you are on a course of study relating to NVQs in Health and Care in general.

Whichever way you choose to use this book, it has been designed to help you by providing information and facts, questions to think about, and links to your experience and practice. Each chapter has been designed to do this by including the following Reader Features.

At the start of each chapter . . .

- Links to NVQ units. At the start of each chapter there is a list of units relevant to the topics covered.
- List of Key Issues.

Within each chapter . . .

You will find a number of boxes which contain questions and give you an opportunity to reflect upon and contemplate issues raised. These include:

- **Think About** points where you are asked to pause and reflect upon your own feelings or experiences.
- **Practice Points** which direct you toward opportunities to consider how your skills and practice might develop in the light of what you have learned.

At the end of each chapter...

- Suggestions for **Further Reading** and **Useful Addresses** which give you the opportunity to explore topics further if you wish.
- **Key terms** – in all specialist subjects a private language tends to develop and so some chapters include a **Glossary** of terms to clarify the terminology used.

At the end of the book, you will find **Appendices** which include helpful guidance on many aspects of studying and presenting evidence of competence, including projects and portfolios. You may be familiar with some of this material, but we hope that you will find it useful as either an update or reminder.

Overall, we hope this volume will provide you with a stimulating foundation on which to build your own skills and develop competence.

Editor's note

Throughout the book, the term "client" has been used to refer to the person being cared for. We have chosen this word, rather than patient because the latter term is usually associated with a recipient of *hospital* care. As a support worker, you may be working in all kinds of areas, many of which are not in hospital.

SECTION

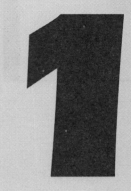

Foundation to care

Introduction

Much to most people's suprise, the Support Worker in Care is not exactly a new idea. This section begins by looking at a brief outline of how the role of support workers has evolved and developed.

Support Workers today are essential and integral members of Health care provision, and their role will continue to change and evolve alongside the changes taking place within health care and the social structure.

It was as part of the changes taking place some years ago that a system was set up to enable people to have their skills recognized, and to encourage people to develop knowledge and understanding about their jobs. This system, known as National Vocational Qualifications, is described in a straightforward manner in an effort to overcome much of the confusion and mystique which so often surrounds them.

You may already be working toward an NVQ or perhaps be considering doing so. Either way the explanations given should help you become familiar and comfortable with the system and the language.

The final part of this section is designed to encourage you to make the most of opportunities that arise in your everyday life. We hope it will help you to think more constructively about how YOU learn, and that learning as an adult can be fun and exciting, thereby helping you to become more confident and competent.

1 | The evolution of support worker training

Aileen Richardson and Kathleen Wheatley

The historical background (Figure 1.1)

A The historical background of caring looks primarily at the practice of medicine. In ancient Egypt, India and Greece medical men were seen as great academic scholars and held in high esteem, as being the only people who had knowledge or education. They had a very privileged position.

B Hippocrates laid the foundations of modern medicine, based on disordered body functions. The majority still considered disease to result from the wrath of the gods and this idea prevailed for many centuries. Superstition was rife and this inhibited progress in the promotion of healthy living.

C The development of Christianity led to care for the sick and weak by the provision of "hospitality" under the auspices of religious orders.

D The dissolution of the monasteries by Henry VIII in the sixteenth century, when he broke away from Rome and founded the English church under his own authority, had a major impact on any further development of Christian caring communities in England. The effect of this was to make local communities, which ultimately became parishes with boundaries, responsible for care of their sick and poor.

E Local taxes funded workhouses for the unemployed poor, with an infirmary for the pauper sick of the Parish. Needless to say, lack of funding meant that provision of care was of very poor quality, and only the desperate and destitute would enter the workhouse.

F When "voluntary hospitals" began to appear, people were required to contribute financially towards their health care. This meant that only those who had some form of income or insurance would receive hospital care. Most of the sick were kept at home. Children, elderly and the terminally ill were tended by the women of the household. Nursing up to this point had not been clearly defined, and charitable organizations staffed their wards with women who were prepared to work in return for very basic food and lodging.

Florence Nightingale was the first to look at nursing as a science, and the research she undertook formed the foundation of health education and promotion as we know it today. "The Hospital should Do the sick no harm" is perhaps

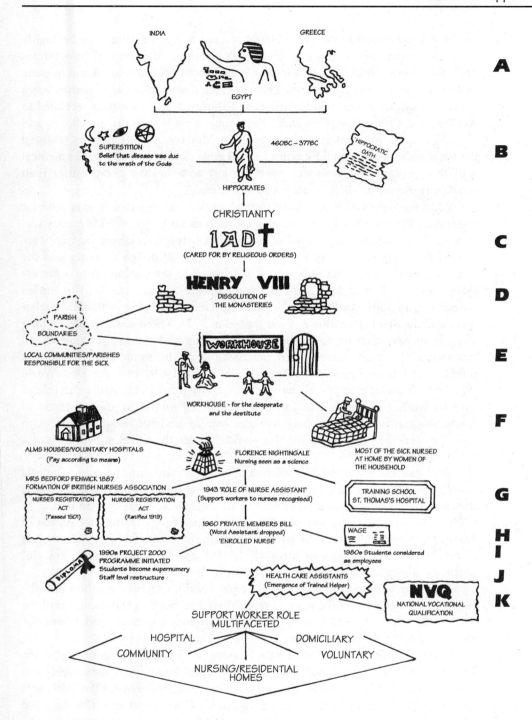

Figure 1.1   The evolution of support worker training

the best known quotation on standards of care and it continues to be highly relevant. As part of her research, Florence's scientific discovery of how micro-organisms were spread had a major impact on standards of sanitation and hygiene in hospitals and in the community. This understanding of disease *prevention* was a major contribution of her work during the Crimean War. The nurses recruited to work in the Crimea spent much of their time scrubbing walls and floors and keeping the environment as clean as possible. Military or army doctors resented the presence of women, and Florence needed great skill in persuading the medical staff that preventative measures were the key to a healthy army rather than medical treatment of disease once it had occurred.

After the Crimean War, a large sum of money was donated in gratitude for the service Florence had given in caring for the sick and injured. This money was used to fund the training school at St Thomas's Hospital, where women were trained primarily to go on to train others elsewhere. Although Florence laid the scientific base to nurse training, she was opposed to the setting up of a professional register. It was Mrs Bedford Fenwick who formed the British Nurses Association in 1887, leading to a Nurses Legislation bill being put before parliament and the first registration Act was passed in 1901. There was thereafter a long struggle to have nursing controlled by a governing body and to provide a legal framework in which nurses could practise and at the same time protect the public. The Nurses Registration Act was ratified in 1919, after the First World War, but no major changes to the Act were made until 1943, when the role of support worker to nurses was formally recognized in law by the provision of Nurse Assistants. These support workers had to undergo examinations with regard to specific practical skills, and worked under the direct supervision of a registered nurse.

A private member's Bill in 1960 had as its main provision the removal of the word "assistant" from the title of Enrolled Nurse. At this time the Enrolled Nurse training and examination system altered to include a written examination in addition to a practical assessment. The next major change to the preparation of nurses for enrolment was in the late 1960s. Hitherto Enrolled Nurse training had primarily been undertaken in hospitals for the elderly and in small "cottage" hospitals, under the direction of a Pupil Nurse Teacher.

Although evolutionary changes took place within nurse education and the examination system over the next 20 years, there was nothing significant until the mid 1980s when the whole structure of nurse education came under scrutiny. This came to be known as Project 2000 (see below).

There had been disquiet within the nursing profession for a number of years. Student status was questioned. Students were considered employees, received a salary, and were subject to the rules and regulations of employment law. Although they were learning they were an essential part of the workforce. Conflicts did arise between educational needs and the need to have nursing staff on the wards. Learners had to shoulder a great deal of responsibility which was often beyond their level of competence. This created a great deal of anxiety and stress, causing many students to leave training.

To enable Project 2000 to be implemented, hospital authorities had to consider how they would provide direct care nursing staff for their wards and departments. Student nurses contributed between 20% and 60% of the care given in hospital wards. The introduction of new-style education and training for nurses meant that there would be a need for carers with a sufficient range of skills to cover the shortfall in staffing levels as learner nurses were withdrawn **J** from the wards. This led to a major review of care staff to identify the number of nurses needed and the number and type of support workers who could assist them in the delivery of care.

The most notable of these surveys was *But Who Will Make The Beds?* (Ball et al. 1990). This work clearly identifies the high percentage of direct personal care given by student nurses and auxiliary grades, and the non-nursing duties which could be undertaken by clerical, domestic and housekeeping staff. Interestingly, prior to Project 2000 there were approximately 112 000 nursing auxiliaries.

Given that the National Health Service could not afford to replace all learners with qualified staff, the idea of a trained helper emerged. These helpers are now known as Health Care Assistants. This coincided with a government initiative to **K** introduce a system of training and assessment programmes to identify competence in fulfilling a known work role. These are the National Vocational Qualifications, described in Chapter 2.

From this brief historical review you can see that the concept of a support worker is not new. What *is* new, however, is the clear identification of the role and educational framework, along with a national recognition of a qualification in care.

Support workers in the health care team

It should not be assumed that the support worker role refers only to the hospital environment. Support workers are needed throughout the care sector. Figure 1.2 shows the range of settings in which support workers are employed outside hospitals.

Some of the areas where a support worker is an integral member of a caring team include:

- Community care
- Physiotherapy
- Chiropody
- Speech therapy
- Children and adults with a disability
- Domiciliary care
- Occupational therapy
- Residential care

Community Nurses (formerly known as District Nurses) are supported by men and women who have their own case load, giving care and assistance to people in their own homes. This enables people with a wide range of disabilities to continue to live in the community.

Physiotherapists are supported by trained helpers who supervise a range of physical activities, both in hospital and in the community. The support worker also has an important role in assisting the Occupational Therapist. Section 4 looks at these areas in more detail. Chiropodists have recently incorporated

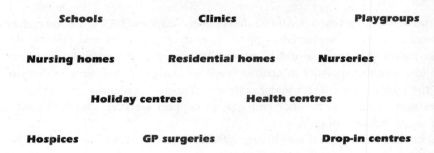

Schools   **Clinics**   **Playgroups**

Nursing homes   **Residential homes**   **Nurseries**

Holiday centres   **Health centres**

Hospices   **GP surgeries**   **Drop-in centres**

Figure 1.2   The wide range of settings for non-hospital support workers

trained foot care assistants into their teams to provide a much needed service to enable people to keep their feet healthy.

Patients these days are being discharged from hospital at an earlier stage following treatment. Social Services have responded by developing the range of skills of "home helps" to enable them to provide care for clients on discharge. Sometimes the help is focused on caring for children of the client, such as taking them to school and seeing to their hygiene needs. In the case of a client living alone they help with financial and nutritional needs by collecting pensions, paying bills, and getting in food.

Support workers are employed to provide a night sitting service, to enable a person or family caring for a sick relative to go out or get a good nights' sleep. The support worker here can be called upon to provide a range of direct care as well as giving psychological support to the family.

The armed forces have always had a large number of support workers in their caring teams. Some are specially trained to give emergency care in the field, as well as for ambulance duties, both in the air and on the ground. They learn how to reach injured personnel in difficult terrain, and survival techniques for adverse weather conditions.

In the realm of learning disabilities, the support worker is concerned with enabling clients to live independent lives and develop social skills, whilst ensuring that they are not taken advantage of by the more fortunate in society. With this client group the support worker can demonstrate the application of all the skills described in the O unit of the NVQ in care.

Support workers are an integral part of many voluntary organizations such as the Red Cross, Order of St John and the Salvation Army. They work alongside professionals, at home and abroad, in a wide range of activities.

REFERENCE

Ball J.A., Hurst, K., Booth, M.R. and Franklyn, R. (1989). *But Who Will Make The Beds?:*, Mersey RHA and the Nuffield Institute for Health Service Studies (University of Leeds).

National Vocational Qualifications

2

Kathleen Wheatley

Vocational qualifications are awarded to people for competent performance at work. NVQs/SVQs were established following a review by a government working party which, in 1986, concluded that only 40% of the working population in Britain held qualifications which were relevant to their job. It was also found that, although a wide range of qualifications were available, many of them bore little or no resemblance to the real world of work. Employers were finding it difficult to recruit staff with skills which would enable them to perform to a high standard without further training. Another problem existed in differentiating between qualifications which were of value and those which were simply a paper exercise.

It was deemed necessary to review the whole structure of education and training. Employers and professionals were invited by the National Council for Vocational Qualifications (NCVQ) in England and Wales, and by the Scottish Vocational Education Council (SCOTVEC) in Scotland, to form Lead Bodies to participate in formulating standards for their particular areas of work. The occupational standards would then be used as the criteria against which candidates (employees) would be assessed, the candidates providing evidence of knowledge, understanding and – above all – competent performance at work.

Levels

NVQs/SVQs, then, are about *assessment at work* in contrast to training and written examinations which, until the introduction of NVQs, were the method of gaining qualifications. Following satisfactory assessment, candidates are awarded the NVQ/SVQ at a level between 1 and 5 according to their work role (see Table 2.1).

NVQs/SVQs are now available in a wide range of occupations throughout industry and commerce, covering work roles and responsibilities from assistant to manager. However, few occupations have developed standards at all five levels. For example, the Operating Department Practitioner's NVQ is awarded at Levels 2 and 3, whereas the Clinical Psychologist is at Level 5. This reflects the particular skills and responsibilities for their current work practice.

Table 2.1 NVQs are awarded at levels 1–5

Level	Work role/responsibilities
1	Areas of work which are repetitive, routine or predictable Foundation skills, generally requiring supervision
2	Work activities which require a larger amount of responsibility from the employee, generally demanding a wider range of skills
3	Areas of skill which are more complex, where activities may not be routine Usually applied to occupational responsibilities which involve supervision of others
4	Skills relating to professional or technical areas which are complex Generally applied to senior supervisory or management levels
5	Highly technical or specialist skills Applies to those with organizational responsibility, at policy-making level

NVQs in care are awarded at Levels 2 and 3. Standards at Level 4 are being identified by the Occupational Standards Counci for Health and Social Care and should be available in the future.

The Lead Body and the Awarding Bodies

The Occupational Standards Council for Health and Social Care (formerly known as the Care Sector Consortium) is the Lead Body responsible for writing the standards for care and work in consultation with the three Awarding Bodies (see Figure 2.1). An Awarding Body is a group or organization approved by the NCVQ or SCOTVEC to issue awards. The three bodies are:

- City and Guilds of London Institute (C&G)
- Central Council for Education and Training in Social Work (CCETSW)
- Business and Technology Education Council (BTEC)

Initially these worked together and were known as a Joint Awarding Body (JAB). Currently the JAB consists of just two bodies, C&G and CCETSW. However, BTEC continues to offer NVQs in care and it is possible that other agencies will become Awarding Bodies in the future.

Obtaining your qualification

By achieving an NVQ/SVQ in care, and working to the standards, you can ensure that your clients receive the best possible care. To achieve an NVQ/SVQ at Level 2 or Level 3 you will have to prove that you can carry out your role to meet the

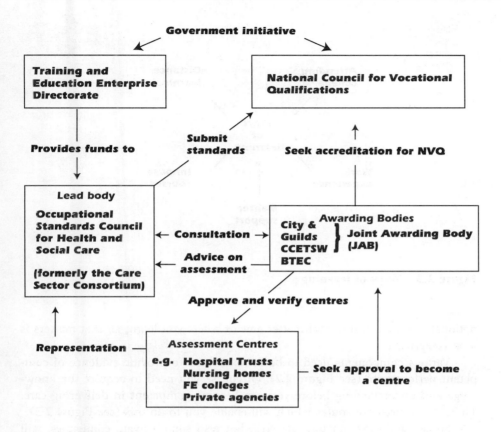

Figure 2.1   The development of NVQs in care

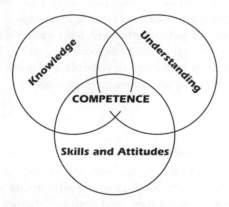

Figure 2.2   Elements of competence

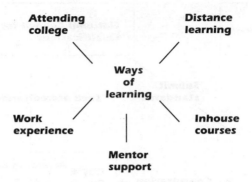

Figure 2.3   Ways of learning

national standard. It does not matter *how* or *where* you learn; all that matters is your *competence*.

Various components need to be demonstrated to provide evidence of competent performance (see Figure 2.2). Of course you need to acquire the knowledge and understanding before you can become competent in delivering care. There are a variety of routes which will enable you to do this (see Figure 2.3).

Some employers, notably the NHS but also some private companies, will provide inhouse courses, or pay for you to attend off-the-job study days and workshops. Others, particularly organizations which employ small numbers, may find it more beneficial for you to attend a local college, or learn through distance-learning packages such as the ones offered by the Open College.

In order to achieve an NVQ/SVQ you must register with one of the Awarding Bodies for your area of employment. Your employer will help you to do this. You will be linked with a qualified mentor/assessor, usually someone with whom you work (e.g. your manager/supervisor, or if you are in a hospital, a staff nurse). Your mentor/assessor is also the person who will help you through the process of learning and practising, to enable you to become competent. If you are attending a course of study your tutor may come to your place of work to give support and guidance through the learning and assessment process.

NVQs/SVQs in care

The standards were written by people from within the care sector, including representatives from the NHS, local government, private care organizations, voluntary organizations, trade unions, and statutory bodies such as CCETSW and City and Guilds.

To achieve your NVQ/SVQ you will need to know about and understand the Occupational Standards for your area in care, and demonstrate through assessment at work that you are competent in carrying out your work to the level described in the written criteria.

Initially, you may find the language in which the standards are written difficult to understand. Try not to worry too much about this, as your mentor/ assessor will help you to relate the standards to your everyday work. It will soon become clear how you can demonstrate your competence within your role in caring.

Sections 2, 3 and 4 of this book have been designed to provide information to support competent practice at NVQ Levels 2 and 3 in care. The book is not about one particular standard or competence, but aims to cover a range of roles and competencies.

To guide you, specific units are identified at the beginning of each chapter. Some units occur frequently, particularly the O Unit as this is central to all your care in any setting.

More about the standards

You will find it useful to know how the standards are constructed. This will help you to identify where they fit in with the everyday work. The standards are divided into **units**. Each unit is about a specific contribution that you make within a whole range of care. For example, the Z *units* are about supporting clients' independence, whilst the X *units* are about supporting clients receiving specific treatments.

Example

You are caring for a client who has suffered a stroke. As part of your role you are required to ensure that the client is provided with adequate food and fluid. The unit which would state the standards are found in:

Unit Z10 – *Enable clients to eat and drink*

The unit title describes the **skill area**.

Elements

The units are then divided into **elements**. The element title describes what you have to do within the skill area.

Performance criteria

Performance criteria describe how you can show, within your normal daily work, that you are applying your knowledge and understanding in dealing competently with the clients' needs.

Example

Going back to the example of Unit Z10, this has three elements, *a*, *b* and *c* (see Figure 2.4). Element *a* has *eight* performance criteria which have to be met to demonstrate your knowledge,

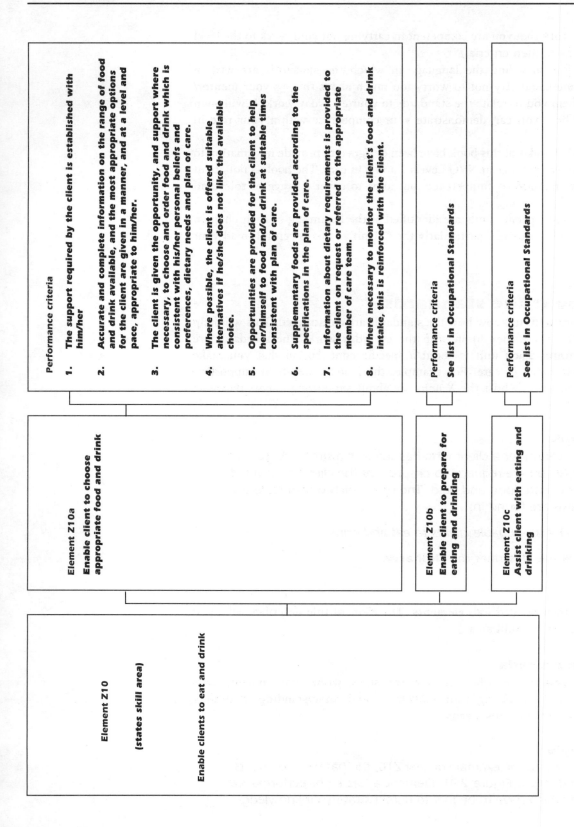

Performance criteria

1. The support required by the client is established with him/her

2. Accurate and complete information on the range of food and drink available, and the most appropriate options for the client are given in a manner, and at a level and pace, appropriate to him/her.

3. The client is given the opportunity, and support where necessary, to choose and order food and drink which is consistent with his/her personal beliefs and preferences, dietary needs and plan of care.

4. Where possible, the client is offered suitable alternatives if he/she does not like the available choice.

5. Opportunities are provided for the client to help her/himself to food and/or drink at suitable times consistent with plan of care.

6. Supplementary foods are provided according to the specifications in the plan of care.

7. Information about dietary requirements is provided to the client on request or referred to the appropriate member of care team.

8. Where necessary to monitor the client's food and drink intake, this is reinforced with the client.

Performance criteria

See list in Occupational Standards

Performance criteria

See list in Occupational Standards

Element Z10a
Enable client to choose appropriate food and drink

Element Z10b
Enable client to prepare for eating and drinking

Element Z10c
Assist client with eating and drinking

Element Z10

(states skill area)

Enable clients to eat and drink

Figure 2.4 Example A from the Occupational Standards

understanding and skill in enabling clients to choose appropriate food and drink. These criteria are listed in Example A from
the National Occupational Standards.

The core and endorsement units

Whether working in hospital, in the community or in another care setting, there
are certain functions that all carers have in common. As seen in the O Unit in
Example B (Figure 2.5), all individuals have the right to be treated as an
individual. The National Occupational Standards in care take this into account,
and everyone working towards an NVQ/SVQ in care is required to have the
knowledge, understanding and ability to demonstrate competence in the skill
areas described in what are known as the **core units** (see Table 2.2).

You will see that the units O, Z1, U4 and U5 appear in both Level 2 and Level
3 cores. If you have achieved an NVQ/SVQ at Level 2 in care you will not have to
repeat these units for Level 3 – with the exception of the O Unit, which has to be

> **Think about**
> Refer to Example A of
> the National
> Occupational Standards
> shown in Figure 2.4.
> What do you think
> could be included in the
> performance criteria for
> element Z10b?

Table 2.2 Core Units

Unit	Level 2	Unit	Level 3
O	Promote equality for all individuals	O	Promote equality for all individuals
Z1	Contribute to the protection of individuals from abuse	Z1	Contribute to the protection of individuals from abuse
W2	Contribute to the ongoing support of clients and others significant to them	Z3	Contribute to the management of aggressive and abusive behaviour
W3	Support clients in transition due to their care requirements	Z4	Promote communication with clients where there are communication difficulties
U4	Contribute to the health and safety of individuals and their care environment	Z8	Support clients when they are distressed
U5	Obtain, transmit and store information relating to the delivery of a care service	U5	Obtain, transmit and store information relating to the delivery of a care service
		U4	Contribute to the health and safety of individuals and their care environment
		Y2	Enable clients to make use of available services and information

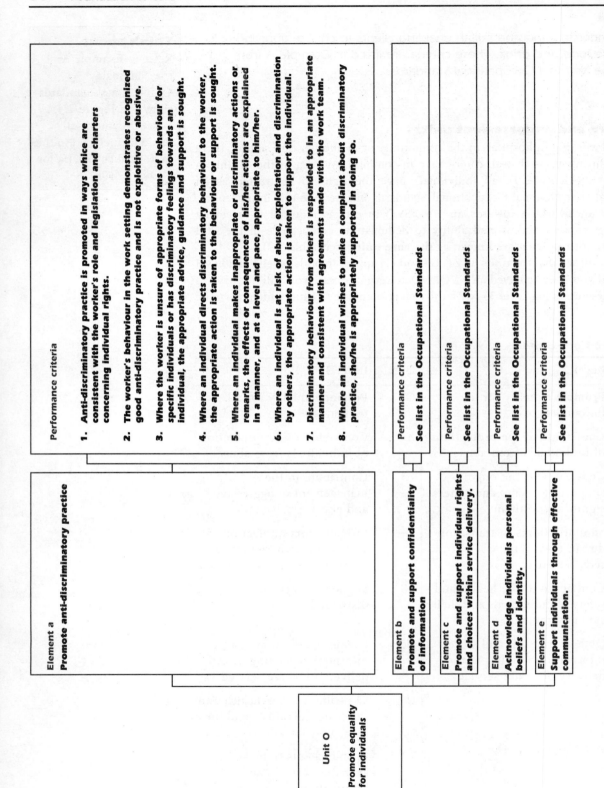

Figure 2.5   Example B from the Occupational Standards

demonstrated in all your caring in whatever capacity you are working. Whilst all other units achieved are transferable, the O Unit is not.

To achieve a full NVQ/SVQ you will need to demonstrate your competence not only in the core units but also in a specific **endorsement unit**.

Example

If you are currently working in the field of mental health you could choose to be assessed in the endorsement units for that area. At Level 3 these are:

Z2   Contribute to the provision of advocacy for clients

X2   Prepare and provide agreed individual development activities for clients

X16   Prepare and implement agreed therapeutic group activities

W1   Support clients in developing their identity and personal relationships

W5   Support clients with difficult or potentially difficult relationships

W8   Enable clients to maintain contacts with potentially isolating situations

Should you change your employment in the future, it is possible for you to do additional endorsement units without having to repeat the core units (with the exception of the O Unit which, as already stated, must be repeated no matter how many other qualifications are undertaken).

Unit credits

It is not necessary for you to achieve a full NVQ/SVQ in a specific period of time. You may choose to do only the units which you (or your employer) think are relevant to your current work role. By providing evidence of competence in all elements of a unit, **unit credits** (certificates of competence for single or multiple units) can be achieved individually and kept to provide evidence, should you decide to work towards a full NVQ in the future.

Assessment and your assessor

As NVQs/SVQs are about competence at work, most assessments will be carried out as part of your normal routine. There will be no formal written examinations, but your assessor will ask you questions about what he or she has seen you do and how you have interacted with clients, relatives and work colleagues. You may be asked to write about it, or to complete a project. The role of your assessor is to ensure that you have provided sufficient evidence to prove your knowledge, understanding and ability to carry out your work to the stated performance criteria for each element and to identify gaps in your knowledge where training is necessary. He or she will need proof that the evidence you provide is all your own work, that there is a wide enough range of evidence to prove competent performance, and that the evidence is up to date and is your current level of competence.

Your assessor will have to show that he or she has assessed you against the written criteria and applied the National Standards in assessment practice, to ensure that all assessments are fair and reliable. A person called an Internal Verifier will in turn need to be satisfied that the assessor is fulfilling his or her role competently. This is to ensure that the standards are being upheld and that you have been given every opportunity to demonstrate your competence.

Most assessments will be undertaken by direct observation of you caring for clients, and participating within a caring team. Your assessment should as far as possible be part of your normal work, but sometimes your assessor, or you, may decide that you can best demonstrate your competence through simulations or role play.

You should have assigned to you by your manager an assessor who has a work-based assessor's qualification. The assessor will be responsible to a senior person for ensuring that all assessments have been agreed and planned with you prior to assessment taking place, and that you have been given adequate opportunity to learn and practise in your work place. There are no time limits set by the National Council for Vocational Qualifications. However, your employer may set some time constraints within your employment contract. It is important that you keep control of the evidence which you collect to demonstrate that you have achieved competence in each and every unit. The section on preparing a portfolio in Appendix I will help you with this.

Points to remember

- NVQs/SVQs are awarded for competence at work.
- NVQs/SVQs are made up of a stated number of units.
- Each unit has a number of elements.
- Each element has a number of performance criteria.
- You must provide evidence that you can meet all the criteria in a unit for a unit credit, and in all the units for a full NVQ/ SVQ.
- The O Unit must be demonstrated within *every* unit.

Preparing for learning

3

Aileen Richardson

The previous chapter has outlined the NVQ system, in particular the NVQs in care. At first you may find the system somewhat confusing, but once you become familiar with the various components you will be able to relate them to your own work area. One of the most important aspects of working towards any qualification is to have knowledge and understanding before applying any skill. *In a nutshell, you need to learn*.

This chapter is about how you as an adult learn and how you can use your **past experiences** to the best advantage. It also covers styles of learning and some specific hints as to how you might improve or develop **study skills**. All these aspects are important, not only for those who are undertaking a specific course of study but for everyday life.

We live in a world of accelerating change. Learning must be a lifelong process, but it need not be dull. *Learning can be FUN*.

Throughout our lives learning continues and is very much a part of life itself. We learn as part of our work, our social roles and relationships, as we enter either new ones or reinterpret existing ones. And we learn anew as we enter new phases of self-development, as we acquire new interests or discover new talents within ourselves. The ultimate goal of this learning is enhanced adulthood, greater maturity and self-development, a fuller sense of perspective, and increased responsibility for ourselves and perhaps for others.

Most of us will perhaps feel that the learning we achieved at school was "compulsory", and associated mainly with passing exams. One of the problems with this type of learning is that it can be difficult to relate the subjects taught to what we want to do with our future. All too often the motivation for learning came from external sources, such as getting good grades or pressure from the teachers and our parents.

To a large extent, learning as a child is directed by others, whereas learning as an adult can become much more *self-directed*. In reading this book you are directing yourself to learn things which relate directly to your work or course.

There are numerous differences between how a child learns and how an adult learns (Knowles 1989). By thinking about how you learn you will not only help yourself to develop but can also use this knowledge to help teach others,

> **Think about**
> Look back on your life and think about how, where and what you have learnt. Was it easy to learn at school? Was it much easier to learn about a subject which interested you?

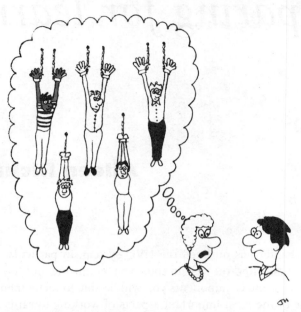

MOTIVATION FOR LEARNING – WELL WITH MY METHODS OF
TEACHING I CERTAINLY HAD NO PROBLEMS.
YES I WOULD SAY MY STUDENTS WERE MOTIVATED, THEY COULD
NOT WAIT TO MOVE ON TO GREATER THINGS.

whether it be clients or their families. Think about the following points and consider how they relate to you.

Adults need to know why they need to learn something before undertaking to learn it

Example

Monica is working in a care setting looking after a number of elderly people. She attends a lecture on fire hazards and reads the policy on fire procedures. She makes certain to learn what she needs to because she realizes that people may suffer if she is not knowledgeable and competent about fire safety.

This illustrates that adults are more able to recognize the relationship between learning and its application to real life, and conversely less prepared to learn something if there is no good reason – unless of course you want to appear on *Mastermind*, although that in itself may be a reason!

Most adults like to feel that they have a responsibility for their own decisions and for their lives

Adults who enrol for Further Education courses do so because they wish to take responsibility for themselves by developing an interest or to improve their career prospects.

Interestingly, perhaps as a result of receiving a more traditional method of schooling, these people tend to sit back and expect to be "taught". This can create conflict in that the adult part of the person rebels against what they believe to be the passive role of the learner. *Learning is not a passive activity*, and to gain the most from learning the adult must participate fully.

Think about
Have you ever heard yourself or others say "But it has always been done that way"? How have others reacted when you tried to change something?

Simply by being an adult, you have a greater volume and different quality of experience from that of children
You will not have had the same experiences at 14 that you will have had by age 35.

In any group of adults the richest resources for learning are within the adults themselves. Put a group of adults together and the combined resources are great.

The other side of the coin is, however, potentially a negative one. As we mature and build up our knowledge and experiences, we also develop biases, habits and presuppositions which tend to create barriers to new ideas, fresh perceptions and thinking in broader terms. Perhaps this is where the saying "You can't teach an old dog new tricks" comes from.

Franz Kafka, in his celebrated short story *Metamorphosis*, produced the aphorism "It is safer to be in chains than to be free." This highlights that by not expanding and opening up your mind you will remain restricted by the chains of your present knowledge and experiences. For many people this is the safest and most comfortable of positions, but it can be rather boring and restrictive.

Motivation for learning

Motivation is perhaps the most crucial aspect of learning. We tend to be motivated to learn new things by the extent to which we see it helping us to perform tasks or deal with problems we confront in our lives. New knowledge, understanding, skills, values and attitudes are most effectively learnt when presented in the context of real life situations.

To a large extent this is encompassed in the philosophy of the NVQ framework. The learning relates directly to real life and the work place.

Example
Elaine was a 38-year-old mother of two children. Both children were adept at using a computer and had tried to encourage their mother to learn the necessary skills. Elaine spent hours reading the computer manual, which started off by asking her to memorize the commands. She found that she forgot them very quickly. It occurred to Elaine that she was trying to learn something for its own sake without knowing *how* she would use it to perform the tasks she wanted the computer to perform.

Elaine wanted to use the computer to write formal letters. She was in the process of applying for a number of jobs, so she ignored the manual and set about teaching herself how to

Think about

Think about five skills
you have acquired or
things you have learnt
in the past five years.
They might include
such things as learning
a foreign language,
knitting, painting,
hanging wallpaper, or
changing a plug. Now
think of the reasons *why*
you learned them. Try
to remember *how* you
learned them.

make the computer format her letters. By relating the learning
to something that was relevant and useful, Elaine rapidly developed her computing skills – much to the surprise of her
children.

Possibly the most powerful motivator to learning comes from the self – the
desire for increased job satisfaction, self-esteem and quality of life.

Your attitude to learning may well be coloured by past experiences, and so
you may love it or hate it! Most people's feelings lie somewhere in between.
Learning should not be thought of as always being structured, and you might be
surprised at how much you have learned informally and through your own and
other's experiences.

The skills and knowledge you have acquired will have been gained for a
variety of reasons and in a variety of ways. You may have learnt to drive because
you needed a car to get to work, and from there you learnt to change a wheel. You
may have learnt a foreign language because you wanted to be able to talk to
people while on holiday abroad.

Life experiences

Learning from life is one of those processes which is easy to take for granted, but
this learning from experience is both important and valuable. Our very person-
alities are moulded by experiences of various kinds. Our skills, beliefs, attitudes
and emotions have evolved, developed and been updated through a process of
trial and error, but this learning from experience needs to be more organized and
conscious.

- How easy was it for you to answer the questions about *how* and *why*
  you learnt your five identified skills?
- Did you acquire these skills all at once or did you learn them gradually
  in stages?

You may have found that task quite easy as you were asked about *skills*; but
how easy is it to answer the following questions?

- What have you done today?
- What have you learnt from what you have done today?
- How did you learn from what you have done today?

This might be more difficult as most people learn from experience in a very
haphazard way. When everything is going smoothly we tend to be rather
complacent and believe that our learning is *instinctive*. When something goes
wrong the complacency is shattered – learning is painful but becomes more
conscious. At other times we may look back on an event and learn from
hindsight, or deliberately try out new and different ways of doing things.

One way of understanding and becoming more efficient at learning from experience is to recognize our learning style preferences. So let us look at the stages that are involved in learning from experience and then at the styles which affect our use of these stages.

1. Having an experience

There are two ways of having an experience. One is to sit back and wait for the experience to come to you, and the other is deliberately to seek it out. The opportunities to learn are greatly increased if we can create extra experiences.

> ### Example
> Mark was escorting one of his clients to the hospital for a routine chest X-ray. Instead of leaving his client with the radiographer he asked if he could remain with his client. Suitably attired in protective clothing, Mark was able to use this opportunity to ask questions about radiography and provide his client with additional support.

2. Reviewing the experience

It is important to think about the experience and consider what has happened. Sometimes the hurly-burly of life takes over and you find you have not reviewed one experience before the next one starts. Your time management skills should help you to pause constructively and think about what is happening. You can develop a **reviewing habit**, which can be done alone, or with others, in about five minutes flat!

> In the example, Mark will be able to think back on his experience. The next time a client requires an X-ray he will be able to reassure and provide accurate information for the client.

3. Drawing conclusions from the experience

How often do you "jump to conclusions"? There is little point in making a conclusion unless you have given a little time to reviewing the experience.

> For Mark, his experience made him realize that many of his own fears around the complex technology of radiography had been unjustified, and perhaps his fears had been transmitted to his clients in the past.

4. Planning the next steps

There would be little point in reaching a conclusion if we did not strive to do something better, or differently, as a result. "Planning" means considering the conclusion and developing an **action plan**.

> Mark decided that he needed to gain more information about radiology, not only for his own benefit but also to be able to give correct information to his clients. He asked questions of the relevant people and was guided to appropriate reading material. Mark used this experience in a positive way rather than letting it slip away as part of the day's activity.

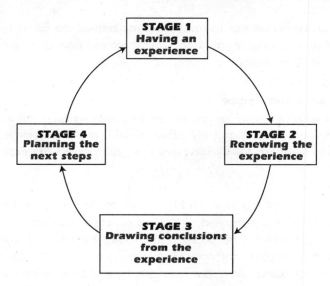

Figure 3.1 The learning cycle

These four stages are interlinked – each stage is of little value in isolation. The whole process is illustrated in Figure 3.1.

Styles of learning

Figure 3.1 may appear quite simple, but many people perform only some parts of the process, as they have unconsciously developed some learning styles which equip them better for certain stages in the cycle than for others (Honey 1989).

The ideal would be to have an even distribution of all four styles, to qualify

> **Think about**
>
> What type of learner are you?
> ▷ An *activist* says "I'll try anything once."
> ▷ A *reflector* says "I'd like time to think about this."
> ▷ A *theorist* says "How does this fit with that?"
> ▷ A *pragmatist* says "How can I apply this in practice?"

as an all-round learner. In reality the majority of people have one or two preferred styles. Perhaps the best way to learn how to learn from experience is to discipline yourself to completing all four stages in the learning cycle shown in Figure 3.1.

You can consider keeping a **learning log** (Open College 1992). This may take you as little as 15 minutes, but you need to be realistic about how often this is possible. The more often the better, but even once a week will be of value. The routine for the log is simple:

■ Think back over a particular experience and pick out the part which had most significance for you. Write down in your own words the details of the particular event or activity.

- Next list any conclusions you reached. Do not worry about the number or practicalities of this, as these are in fact your learning points.
- Finally, decide which learning points you want to do something about, and make a plan as to how and when you will achieve them. *You need to be realistic*, the learning needs to be achievable. If you set the goals too high you will be discouraged when you cannot achieve them.

This process of self-discipline will help you get the most out of all your experiences.

Getting ready to learn

Now that you have considered your own particular learning style, the next step is to consider how you might develop your style and improve your study skills. Remember that learning and acquiring new skills is an ongoing process.

You may be starting to study for the first time in years, or you may have studied regularly for some time. Either way, you should give some consideration as to *how* you study. At the beginning of your studies you need to think carefully about the following points.

Managing your time

This means that you have to *find time* by planning out your week, and *use time* in the most effective way. Appendix I(i) gives you more ideas on this.

Finding somewhere to study

This is not always very easy! You do need to have some space where you can work undisturbed, with room to spread out your books and papers. It is also important that the environment is comfortable, so you need to consider such things as temperature, noise and lighting. You may be able to adapt your home environment in some way, or you might prefer to study in the local library or borrow a quiet spot in a friend's house.

Wherever you study, it helps if you tell people that you do not want to be disturbed, and set a time limit for this.

Obtaining equipment

You do not need to buy out the local stationary shop! You need to have pens and notepads, and a system of storing information. The system you use does not matter provided that you can retrieve the information you want, when you want it.

Developing concentration and motivation

This is a vital step. You need to focus your attention on what you are learning and remind yourself frequently of the benefits.

Point to remember

The normal concentration span is only about 20 minutes, so mix reading with writing, thinking and doing. When your concentration wavers then STOP. Take a short break, setting a limit of perhaps 10 minutes. Make a cup of tea, take the dog for a walk or just sit and relax.

There *will* be times when you feel you have lost motivation for studying. The following pointers may help to revive you:

- *Reward yourself* when you have achieved a planned task.
- *Enlist help* from a friend or family member, who will support and encourage you.
- *Get some feedback.* This is vital for maintaining your motivation and giving you confidence. Your tutor, mentor, supervisor and colleagues can all help.
- When you find yourself struggling with a particular task, stop and reconsider your approach. *Is there a better way of doing it?*
- *Define the tasks.* Decide what tasks need doing, and if possible break them down into smaller and more manageable units. By dividing the task into smaller pieces and completing each piece one at a time, you are more likely to complete the whole task (in the same way that you might approach a large jigsaw puzzle).

Example

You need to read a particular book for the following week. Depending on the size and content, divide the book into manageable sections, aiming to read one section each night. By doing this you can then manage your time better.

Points to remember

Learning is a lifelong activity, and although the purpose of studying is to learn, it should also be fun.

- Open up to new ideas, throw off the chains.
- Think through new ideas alongside your existing ones, so building up a better understanding of your subject.
- Practise expressing these new ideas verbally and in writing.
- The appendices in this book give further information on study skills relevant to preparing for an NVQ in care.

Further reading

Freeman (1991), Mastering Study Skills (Macmillan Educational).

Freeman and Meed (1991), How to Study Effectively (National Extension College).

Open University (1990), The Good Study Guide (OU).

REFERENCES

Honey, P. (1989). Article published in the *Guardian*, 19 December.

Knowles, M. (1989). *The Adult Learner: A Neglected Species*, 3rd edn, Gulf Publishing.

Open College (1992). Professional Development Enrolled Nurse Conversion Learning Materials.

SECTION

Healthy living

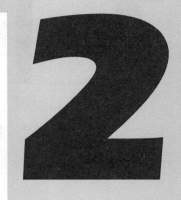

Introduction

This section is about *you*, about *people* and about *health*. In all aspects of health care provision the concept of *holistic care* takes into account the physical, psychological and social needs of the individual. Respect for all individuals is fundamental to the principles of holistic care and must be demonstrated in the care you give. In recognizing individuality, **Chapter 4** explores some ideas on why and how each and every one of us is different.

To develop your understanding of what individuality means, the best place to start is with yourself. Chapter 4 will help you to:

■ identify some aspects of your life which make you the unique person you are
■ identify ways of developing a more positive self-image
■ identify ways of promoting a positive self-image in others.

A positive self-image is one aspect of health, but what does being "healthy" really mean? In **Chapter 5** the factors which affect health and the concept of *health promotion* are discussed. Your role in promoting and maintaining health is identified.

Continuing with the theme of health, **Chapter 6** addresses the issue of *mental health* and considers some psychological issues which you may encounter in any care setting. This chapter provides you with some strategies to help maintain and promote the mental health of your clients.

The last two chapters in this section are about *healthy attitudes*. **Chapters 7 and 8** promote the development of healthy attitudes by dispelling the stereotyped view held by many people, about the elderly and people with learning disabilities.

4 | *A unique individual*

Elizabeth Bulmer

This chapter looks at some aspects of psychological development, and how past experiences can have a positive or a negative effect on subsequent behaviour.

An understanding of these issues will enable you to become more skilful in your dealings with people, taking into account that psychological attributes, social and emotional health are not static. They are affected by the very process of growing older, by illness, by disability and by hospitalization, which in turn makes people vulnerable.

The study of anatomy and physiology is important in learning to care for people, but equally it is important to have some understanding of human behaviour. Care should be **holistic** – including the mind as well as the body – and must recognize individual differences.

Many of the issues discussed here are pertinent to a wide range of people and care situations.

The key issues of this chapter are:
- Understanding people
- Life positions
- Individuality
- Ego-grams

Understanding people

In attempting to understand other people the best place to start is with yourself. Although each and every one of us is unique and very individual, there are some common threads which, if identified, can give insight into other people's feelings and behaviour. Some argue that self-awareness leads to introspection and self-centredness, but this fear is unfounded and indicates a distorted view of self-awareness. In reality it should lead to a deeper understanding of people in general and of how relationships function. It should encourage you to question your own attitudes and prejudices.

This chapter links with units Oa, Oc, Od and Z4 b1, Z4 b8.

This understanding plays a vital role in helping to meet the physical, psychological, social and emotional needs of clients.

There are many books available on both physical and psychological development, which discuss these in great depth. However, this chapter is based on one particularly well-known theory called **transactional analysis** (TA). This was originated by Dr Eric Berne (1910–70).

TA is a theory of personality structure and a method of psychotherapy. "Transaction" refers to the **communication** which takes place between two people. "Analysis" refers to an **investigation** into the feelings and behaviour patterns that are demonstrated during the transaction. Although the theory sounds quite complicated, basically it provides a few pointers into what influences peoples' behaviour.

To gain the most from this chapter you should consider your own behaviour and try to relate it to how other people behave. How we see ourselves and how others see us can often be poles apart because **perceptions** differ. Look at Figure 4.1: in this picture what do you see, an old lady or a young girl?

Just as you may have a false opinion of a person they may equally have a false opinion of you, and this can have an effect on the way you relate to each other.

Self-perception can lead to a false **self-image**. A young girl may consider herself fat even though she is the correct weight for her height and build. Taken to extremes, some girls develop anorexia because they perceive themselves too fat while in reality they are painfully thin.

A girl may feel that she is in control of her life by restricting her diet so severely. However, research has found that people differ as to how they see themselves – some as being in control of their lives and some as passive victims

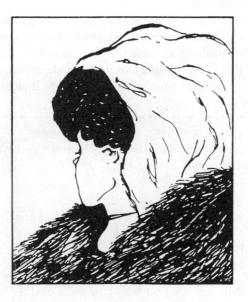

Figure 4.1   What do you see? (after Boring 1930)

Think about
Can you think of anything which has occurred in your past, or a belief you have, which has strongly influenced your behaviour?

of fate. Those who have control have been found to suffer less from depression as a result of illness, and they participate more in their rehabilitation.

If in some way we could understand better what makes people what they are, life would be much clearer and relationships more straightforward. We would have more control over our lives and not be inhibited so much by past experiences and outmoded beliefs.

An historical example of this was the belief that the world was flat and that if you ventured too far you would fall off the edge. The distance people would dare to travel was limited by that belief. Another example might be that if you believe everyone over the age of 70 is deaf you will always shout at people who are elderly.

Developing healthy attitudes

At birth we are totally dependent on parental figures for our survival – if they abandoned us we would die. As babies we soon learn how to attract attention and have our needs and wants met. Our experiences of the most effective methods of getting what we want often continue into adult life, and we adopt stances which remain unless we make conscious decisions to change them.

There are four elementary **life positions:**

I'm OK and you're OK   I'm not OK but you're OK

I'm OK but you're not OK   I'm not OK and you're not OK

We tend not to remain in the same position all the time, but there will be one particular position (or attitude) which we favour.

I'm OK and you're OK

This is a healthy position. In this position we value ourselves and others as human beings, even though at times we may neither agree nor like others' behaviour. In this life position we have the best chance of getting on with people because we realize that compromises have to be made in order to satisfy our own needs without ignoring other peoples'. We set out to look for ways of working and living together.

Think about
Imagine that you and three friends or family members are planning a day out. You have six choices:
  ► Theme park
  ► Seaside
  ► Exhibition
  ► Theatre
  ► Football match
  ► A day's shopping

How do you set about agreeing on where to go? Consider what compromises each of you has to make.

I'm not OK but you're OK

When we are young we soon discover that there are a number of things we cannot do as well as adults. Eating with a knife and fork or tying our shoelaces is difficult. If parental figures repeatedly call us stupid or clumsy as we attempt to learn, then we begin to believe that we are stupid and clumsy and that everyone else is better and brighter.

On being convinced that we are less able than others, there is a temptation to behave in a way such as to reinforce this belief. We then see ourselves as lacking in confidence, and by the way we behave this is communicated to others.

Example

Susan was a young woman who had been unsuccessful in a nursing course final examination and had been working as a nursing auxiliary for a number of years. Susan was encouraged by friends to undertake support worker training but lacked confidence in her written work. This lack of confidence was due largely to Susan's mother reminding her repeatedly of the previous failure. This reinforced Susan's belief that she would always fail when written work was required.

I'm not OK and you're not OK

This is known as the futile position, and when we have had a really bad day this is how life might appear! Some people feel, for a variety of reasons, that they must blame others for their own feelings of pessimism. Their attitude to life is one of hopelessness, believing that nothing or no-one can help or be trusted. This inevitably makes others avoid the person, which in turn reinforces the original belief.

Example

Jane and Sarah were on a training course. Jane was finding the course work very difficult. She had a young family, one of whom was ill, and financial worries added to her problems. Jane became withdrawn and cynical. Sarah tried to find out what was causing Jane's unhappiness, but Jane merely ignored Sarah's offer of help, saying that she would not understand even if she could be bothered to tell her.

I'm OK but you're not OK

In this position we constantly look for faults in other people, in an attempt to justify our own behaviour. This position may be more recognizable to you in children and adolescents in particular. Children often believe that they can do things much better than an adult and that they know better.

However, if this position continues into adult life, the belief that the "I'm OK" person has that he or she is always right will have an adverse effect on relationships with other people. This type of person often appears conceited and overbearing, regularly telling people what they should do and how to do it.

> **Think about**
> Look back at the last week. How often have you made a compromise either at work or at home?

Think about

Reflect on the past week, both at home and at work.

I'm OK and you're OK

Was there a group of people or a particular individual you related well to? If so, what was it about the person or group that helped you to relate to them? Was it because you had something in common, or a shared interest? How well did you relate to all the other people you met?

As a carer you can improve your relationships with a wide range of people by developing your communication skills and by showing a genuine interest in others. This will have a very positive impact not only on those you care for but also with friends and colleagues.

I'm not OK but you're OK

How often did you allow yourself to feel incompetent? Most of us at times will feel that we have not accomplished our duty as well as we should. However, if you regularly feel incompetent this will be reflected in your behaviour and your clients are unlikely to feel confident of your abilities.

This is not unlike a vicious circle and you will continue to feel incompetent unless you break the circle. One way you can do this is by learning the skills needed to become competent in your work role. This in turn will improve your self-image and improve the quality of care you give.

I'm not OK and you're not OK

Did any situations arise which you felt were futile? This can happen, for example, when caring for someone who is trying to come to terms with a terminal illness, in themselves or in a loved one. Anger and a feeling of hopelessness are two of the stages they may go through, and you may feel that anything you say or do for them is futile. Chapter 7 addresses some of these issues in more detail and will help you to cope with such situations.

I'm OK but you're not OK

Did you often feel that you knew better than anyone else? You may have thought "I am a prince and you are a frog!" It is irrelevant whether you did, in fact,

Example

Adrian was a manager. At meetings he would ask his staff for ideas, but when they ventured ideas he would give a patronising and derisory laugh followed by a "Yes, but . . .". He appeared to look down his nose at others, and eventually the staff did not participate in any of these meetings and allowed Adrian to make the decisions. This justified Adrian's belief that he was always right.

Practice point

Once you have given some thought to this, show how much of your time you spent in each life position by drawing a pie chart like the one in Figure 4.2.

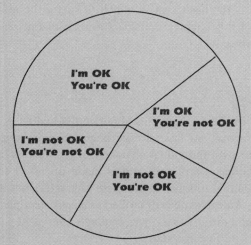

Figure 4.2   A pie chart of life positions

Whilst doing this you may become more aware of your options to spend more time in the healthy position "I'm OK and you're OK". It is important how other people respond to you, and even more so when these people are in one of the "unhealthy" positions.

Being conceited and overbearing will not help you to establish caring and trusting relationships, which are essential if you are to work effectively as a member of a care team. Also, with clients the danger is that you will not allow them to make their own decisions and they will become passive recipients of care. *Developing interpersonal skills, communication skills and being interested in others are all vital in dealing with people.*

Some people are stable in their one position, others move around erratically. By being alert you can recognize which position a person is in and respond appropriately.

Here are some more questions which may help:

- What problems arise at work because of my belief about myself and others?
- What do I believe is the worst thing that might happen if I see myself and others as OK?
- What options do I have for behaving in an "OK" way towards myself and others in specific situations?
- In which situation do I stand the best chance of a successful outcome?
- What do I need to do to spend more time in the healthy position?

We each view the world from a variety of positions. We adopt a position in which we feel comfortable – even though it may not be the healthiest – and we tend to ignore anything which challenges our beliefs. *The life position we choose will dictate our overall attitude to ourselves and others.* Therefore the "I'm OK and you're OK" position is the healthiest in which to spend the most time.

The next part of this chapter, considers aspects of our development which affect our **individuality**.

Individuality

The *Concise Oxford Dictionary* says this about individuality: "separate existence and individual character". So how do we begin to exist separately from our parents and form our own individual character or personality?

Your personality has a structure and is made up of all the characteristics which make an individual unique. In TA these characteristics are known as **ego states** (Berne 1966). An ego state is described as *a consistent pattern of feeling and experience which relates directly to a correspondingly consistent pattern of behaviour* (Berne 1966). There are five ego states:

- Controlling parent
- Nurturing parent
- Adult
- Adapted child
- Natural child

These ego states will be discussed in turn, with some examples given of the behavioural clues to each.

When we are children our parents are **role models** from which we learn our behavioural responses. Our ego states are full of parental influences, the number of which differs for each of us. Some of us may have had just one significant parent figure, others may have had many such as childminders, teachers and grandparents.

We devise our ego states from each of our parental figures.

The controlling parent ego state

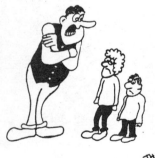

In the controlling parent ego state, the individual behaves, thinks and feels in the same way as the parental figure from the past, when they were establishing rules and being firm.

This ego state is the one we use when we need to be firm and take care of others by setting down rules and boundaries. It can be useful at work to iron out uncertainties by making policies and procedures on how things should be done (e.g. fire procedures and infection control policy).

If we put too much energy into our controlling parent ego state, we could be seen as bossy, overpowering and overcritical of others. Others may get fed up with our ordering them about, and are more likely to rebel than conform. Results based on firmness rather than resentful compliance represent true skill.

Example

Vera, a ward sister, on finding a patient who was confined to bed attempting to get out, shouted loudly "Get back into that bed *immediately*!" She had spoken and sounded like her mother had done when Vera was ill in bed as a child, but on reflection she realized that this was inappropriate when speaking to another adult.

Think about
Have you ever behaved in such a way that someone has commented how like your mother or father you are?

Behavioural clues

Words: ought, should, must, always, never, don't, ridiculous, wicked
Tones: critical, preaching, condescending, aggressive
Gestures and expressions: frowning, pointing finger, accusing gaze, arms folded
Attitudes: judgemental, moralistic, authoritarian
Positive aspects: provides and enforces law, manners, sets limits, traditions
Negative aspects: denies self-worth of others, inflexible, does not allow fun in self or others.

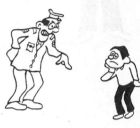

The nurturing parent ego state

In the nurturing parent ego state, the individual behaves, thinks and feels like a parental figure from the past when they were looking after someone and being kind and caring.

We need this ego state at times when caring for others or when looking after someone who is ill. However, over-use of this ego state becomes smothering – it may take over and deny individuals the possibility of developing their skills. That is the negative aspect of the nurturing parent.

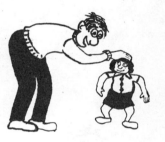

Example

Jamile started work in a small community home helping to care for a number of children who were physically disabled. She loved caring for these children and went to great lengths to do everything she possibly could for them. After a few weeks Jamile, with the help of her supervisor, was able to see that by doing everything for the children she was not allowing them to develop and to learn basic skills for themselves. With support she discovered how to stand back more, and to recognize when to step in and help.

Behavioural clues

Words: good, nice, never mind, there there, I love you, let me help
Voice tone: loving, gentle, comforting, concerned
Gestures and expressions: smiling, open arms, touching others, nodding
Attitudes: understanding, caring, unselfish
Positive aspects: cares and supports others when they want it
Negative aspects: smothering, takes away power from others

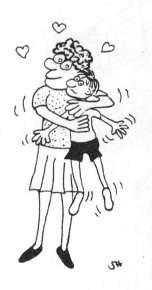

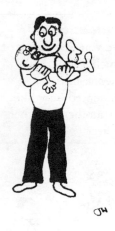

The adult ego state

In the adult ego state, the individual behaves, thinks and feels as an adult does, acting in a logical and problem-solving way.

The adult ego state is not the same as being "grown-up". A child quickly learns that all actions have consequences. A child who drops something from a high chair learns that someone will pick it up. If this is repeated often, the child will recognize anger and irritation from the adult and begin to understand that some form of compromise is needed.

As we grow and develop skills of problem-solving and decision-making, we balance priorities and decide between conflicting requirements. We have to take into account others' feelings as well as our own. Too much time spent being calculating and analytical, however, may make us boring and somewhat of a "cold fish".

Example

This morning your bank statement arrives. You go through the statement with your cheque stubs and work out how much money you have for the rest of the month. This is the adult ego state. It is the here-and-now: being logical and using a problem-solving approach.

It cannot be said that all situations benefit from pure analysis. Sometimes **intuition** may help us make a better decision. If we are *always* logical, we may appear to others like a robot.

Behavioural clues

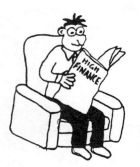

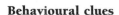

Words: how, what, where, why, appropriate, need, correct, be logical
Tones: even, measured, calm
Gestures and expressions: thoughtful, alert, direct eye contact, attentive
Attitudes: evaluative of facts, dispassionate, objective, controlled
Positive aspects: unbiased, calm, rational, consistent, autonomous
Negative aspects: unfeeling, dull, boring.

The adapted child ego state

In the adapted child ego state, the individual behaves, thinks and feels as a child, when (for example) told to be polite and courteous to others.

Very early on in childhood we learn that doing what we want is not always acceptable to others. Even before we can talk we start to realize – from the way people hold us and by the tone of their voice – that they have expectations of how we should behave. In other words, the **verbal and non-verbal language** of others influences our behaviour and an adapted child ego state develops. No man is an island; therefore individuals need to learn how to fit in, not only with their family but also with society.

There are, however, two extremes. At one extreme, overuse of adapted child behaviour projects an image of a lack of confidence, which may result in our not being trusted with responsibility or decision-making. Additionally, by not refusing inappropriate demands we may be seen as weak and ineffectual.

At the other extreme, we may have learnt in childhood to overcompensate for weakness, appearing aggressive and rebellious. This is also a part of the adapted child ego state. As adults, by doing the exact opposite of what is expected, we are perceived as being awkward and stubborn, and any suggestions we make may be dismissed out of hand, as people think we just want to "start another argument". Rebellion is an adaptation as there is a compulsion to do that rather than choosing how to behave from our own range of options.

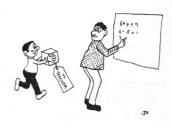

Most people exhibit one extreme or another at certain points in their lives (during teenage years for example), but difficulties arise when one extreme becomes the norm.

Example

Margaret's friend asked whether she would drive her to the airport as she was going away on holiday. However, Margaret's partner had been working abroad and was due home the same evening. Instead of asking her friend to find someone else, Margaret gave in and drove her to the airport, meanwhile resenting the time away from her partner. Margaret reminded herself of all the times when she did things for her father to avoid his anger. She was in her adapted child ego state.

Behavioural clues

Words: I can't, I hope, please, thank you, may I?
Tones: placating, pleading, whiny, muted
Gestures and expressions: innocent, pouting, smiling coyly, eyes lowered
Attitudes: demanding, compliant, subservient, procrastinating
Positive aspects: polite, showing courtesy and respect, eager to please and learn
Negative aspects: self-destructive to get attention, conformist, denies own creativity by having no confidence.

The natural child ego state

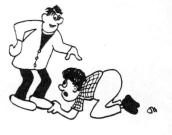

In the natural child ego state, the individual behaves, thinks and feels as a child does, when being spontaneous, friendly and creative.

At birth we have only our natural child ego state. In it we display our genuine feelings – we let people know our needs and act on impulse. As we develop we show our creativity and start to become curious. Children have a huge capacity for friendliness and affection, but as we develop into adults we may curtail our child-like behaviour or be afraid to show it. The acting profession has a saying "Do not work with animals or children", because their natural behaviour can be very disarming!

In our natural child ego state we allow the people we trust to know our genuine happiness, anger or sadness, and we form close relationships as people warm to the fact that they know how we really feel. If, however, we spend too much time in this ego state we may be labelled as childish, immature and silly. People may not believe that we can achieve serious tasks. Our friendliness may be seen as too good to be true and rather "suspect".

It must be said that there are times when it is not appropriate to show our genuine emotions. A managing director has to resist bursting into tears at a board meeting because his dog has died.

Think about

Alone or in a group, brainstorm more behavioural clues for each of the ego states, remembering their positive and negative aspects.

Example

When we are in our natural child ego state we are neither adapting nor rebelling against anyone. We are said to be *spontaneous*. Examples of the natural child ego state are screaming with delight on a fairground ride, reacting like a child to a pantomime, or openly expressing anger if pushed aside in a queue.

Behavioural clues

Words: ouch!, hi!, great, I want, I love, I don't like, lets have fun

Tones: loud, lively, energetic

Gestures and expressions: laughing, grinning, uninhibited, active, spontaneous, unrestrained, wide open eyes, touching and other body contact

Attitudes: fun-loving, joyful, changeable, hurt, vulnerable, sensual, angry, excitable, sexual

Positive aspects: open and direct, fun, joy and pleasure

Negative aspects: destructive of self and others while having fun, selfish.

Ego-grams

In order to discover how important each of the above functional ego states is to ourselves, Jack Dusay devised an intuitive exercise and called it an **ego-gram** (Dusay 1977).

Practice point

Draw a horizontal bar and label it with each of the five main functional ego states (see Figure 4.3)*.

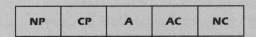

| NP | CP | A | AC | NC |

Figure 4.3

Look back over the past 24 hours and begin by drawing a vertical bar above the ego state label where you feel that you have spent *most* of your time. Now draw a bar over the ego state label where you feel you have spent the *least* of your time. Finally complete the other three bars.

*NP, nuturing parent; **CP**, controlling parent; **A**, adult; **AC**, adapted child; **NC**, natural child.

Example

Denise had been working in the local outpatient department of a general hospital for some years. Being married and with two young children, over the past year Denise had found it increasingly difficult to cope with the hours of work and maintain her home to the standard she liked. This made her very irritable with her work colleagues and her family. She began to realize that most days she had been unsmiling and very brusque with the clients attending the clinics. When she overheard her young daughter tell a friend "Mum really is no fun anymore" she decided to do something about it. Denise's ego-gram at this time would have looked like Figure 4.4.

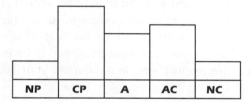

Figure 4.4

On recognizing the need to change her behaviour, Denise considered what her priorities were and how she might change. Managing time better and delegating more of the household tasks was a good start. At work Denise made a conscious effort to listen to others and to be aware of her body language. She soon discovered that when she smiled people reacted in a more positive way. This change in behaviour also had a positive effect on her family life, making it much more fun. After a few weeks Denise's ego-gram looked like Figure 4.5.

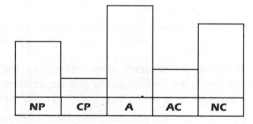

Figure 4.5

You will perhaps by now have realized that understanding human behaviour and individuality is no easy task. It is important always to bear in mind that we are all individuals, and the behaviour of others, and life events, have all played a part in shaping who and what we are. There are no hard and fast rules about

Think about

Is there any particular part of your ego-gram you would like to change? How do you think you might be able to make that change? (Don't forget that your ego-gram may change in different situations, i.e. between work and home.)

Think about
Ask someone who knows you well to do your ego-gram. Does the ego-gram you did for yourself match this one, or do you see yourself very differently from how this other person sees you? Some of you may well find that your perspective of yourself is different from how others view you.

dealing with people, but respect for any other human being is paramount. Respect encompasses the individuals' wishes, choices, decisions and rights.

It would be very difficult in your role as a support worker to attempt to analyse the behaviour of everyone you come into contact with, and it is important to remember that we cannot and should not make presumptions about why someone is behaving in a particular way. But some understanding of our own development and behaviour can be of help in improving the care we give to others. *Providing care is about being able to relate to others and to empathize.*

Conclusion

This chapter has focused on self-awareness, through the theory of transactional analysis. We hope that the points raised will have given you much food for thought. Volumes have been and will continue to be written about the complexities of human development and behaviour and about the variables which influence who we are and what we become. This chapter is not intended to be conclusive nor comprehensive but may encourage you to investigate the psychological aspects which affect your clients and influence your behaviour as a carer.

Points to remember

- Caring for others requires an understanding of human development and behaviour.
- To attain this understanding you should give some thought to the values, beliefs, attitudes and perceptions which you have, and how these may influence your behaviour towards other people.
- The carer should consider ways of developing a positive self-image and promoting a positive self-image in others.
- A positive self-image will lead to positive and confident interactions.

Glossary

Holistic.   Meaning "whole". In the broader context of caring, the individual's physical, emotional and social needs are recognized as interdependent, and he or she is treated as a complete person rather than as the sum of various diseases or needs.

Psychology.   The science dealing with the mind and mental processes, especially in relation to human and animal behaviour.

Psychotherapy.   Any of a number of related techniques for treating mental illness by psychological methods.

Further reading

Stewart and Joines (1987), TA Today (Lifespace Publishing). An informative book on TA which gives lots of exercises to raise self-awareness.

Woollams and Brown (1978), Transactional Analysis (Dexter Hurron Valley Institute).

Levin (1988), Cycles of Power. Explains the cycles of development in full with exercises in correcting needs deficits (Hollywood: C.A. Health Communications).

Hey (1993), Working it out at Work (Sherwood Publishing). Helps the reader understand attitudes and how to build relationships. Julie Hey is clear and practical in her writing and is acknowledged as being of help in the construction of this chapter.

Tschudin and Scober (1990), Managing Yourself (Macmillan).

Paton and Brown (1991), Lifespan Health Psychology (Chapman & Hall).

Jacobs (1992), Sigmund Freud. Describes Freud's life and his major contributions to psychological theory (Sage Publications).

REFERENCES

Berne, E. (1966). *Principles of Group Treatment*, Oxford University Press.

Dusay, J. (1977). *Ego-grams*, Harper and Row.

5 | *Promoting health*

Mike Hemsworth

> . . . in a well run society each man . . . has no time to spend his life being ill and undergoing cures . . . there's nothing worse than this fussiness about one's health . . . it is tiresome in the home, as well as in the army or in any civilian office.   Plato's *The Republic*

In ancient Greece a sound mind and sound body were considered to be the ideal. But can one attain such an ideal? Health is not an absolute quantity but a concept which is continually changing with the acquisition of knowledge and with changing cultural expectations.

This chapter examines the concept of health which relates to the individual and the community. It will provide you with the opportunity to consider the factors which affect health, and the strategies which can be used to promote health. All health care workers have a commitment to the health of individuals, families and the community. The support worker as part of the care team has a role in

- helping individuals to prevent disease and maintain a stable state of health
- helping individuals to modify their behaviour to attain a higher quality of health and life
- helping individuals who are or have been ill to improve their functional ability.

The key issues of this chapter are:
- Defining what is meant by the term "health"
- Understanding the basic concepts of health education, health promotion and the distinction between the two
- Identifying your role in promoting health and providing health education for your clients
- Identifying local, national and international agencies concerned with health, health education and health promotion

This chapter links with units Oc, Od, Y2 and U4.

What is this thing called "health"?

The World Health Organization (WHO) and many other groups have put forward a number of definitions of health. Before we look at these, complete the following exercise which will help you to clarify what health means to you as an individual.

Practice point

Write down the numbers 1 to 16, and tick the numbers of the following statements which you feel are important aspects of health for you. *For me being healthy means*:

1 being physically fit
2 feeling I am getting the most out of life
3 not having any bad habits such as smoking
4 liking myself most of the time
5 being free from disease
6 feeling glad to be alive when I wake up in the morning
7 hardly ever taking medicines
8 being able to adapt easily to the changes in my life
9 being the ideal weight for my height
10 enjoying being with my friends and family
11 hardly ever going to the doctor
12 enjoying some form of relaxation or hobby
13 feeling in harmony with nature and the universe
14 never having a major illness or accident
15 being able to cope with the pressures of life
16 having all the parts of my body in working order.

"Being healthy is not the same as not being ill"

In the past when infectious diseases were the predominant causes of illness and death, health was defined in terms of the *absence of disease*. By the mid-1900s, the incidence of many of these infections had been reduced and health had come to mean more than simply not being ill.

Probably the best known definition of health was issued in 1946 by the World Health Organization as:

   a state of complete physical, mental and social well-being, and not merely the absence of disease or infirmity

When this definition was put forward it was believed that there was a clear distinction between health and ill-health.

When the National Health Service (NHS) was being planned it was assumed that there was a limited number of people who were ill and that once they were treated the annual cost of the health service would be reduced. With the benefit of hindsight we know that health includes more than physical aspects, and much more than the absence of disease. However, the 1946 statement opened the door for discussion about the more positive features of health, and their implications for public policy.

Think about
▷ Are there different beliefs about health even within the same society?
▷ Is it possible for you to be healthy when you are part of a community which is socially deprived?

Over the past 50 years there has been a growing awareness that health must be seen from an individual perspective, dependent on personal and social resources, and the ability to adapt to and cope with the challenges met throughout life.

Someone who *feels* well and lives in a way that he or she finds socially and economically satisfactory may be considered healthy, even with a disease or significant disability. On the other hand, someone with no detectable evidence of physical illness may be judged "unhealthy" because he or she feels unwell.

Health as a human right

Just as health is dependent upon personal and social resources, health is a resource in itself, and gives us the ability to manage and even change our surroundings. It is a basic and dynamic force in our daily lives, influenced by our circumstances, our beliefs, our culture and our social, political, economic and physical environments. It should be considered as an essential human right.

Every individual has a right to grow up in an environment in which there is sufficient food, shelter and mental stimulation to enable him or her to reach full potential. The WHO's statement "Health for all by the year 2000" recognizes that health is a right for people throughout the world.

Further perceptions of health

Consider the following definitions of health.

- ■ "[Health is] a process of adaptation . . . the ability to adapt to changing environments, to growing up and ageing, to healing when damaged, to suffering, and to the peaceful expectation of death." (Illych 1976)
- ■ "Health cannot be possessed, it can only be shared. There is no health without my brother. There is no health for Britain without Bangladesh." (Wilson 1976)
- ■ "Good health is possible if you are able to choose to do a job you enjoy, in a pleasant and safe environment, to live in a warm house with enough space so that people do not get on top of one another, and with a safe place for your children to play, to be able to have your children looked after during the day, eat the food you like best, to have a garden, to live in the country or to be able to get away to the country at weekends. It is having time with people you love and time on your own." (Brent Community Health Council 1985)
- ■ "An individual has health when he possesses a sense of optimum well-being which enables him to lead a personally satisfying and socially useful life." (Anon)
- ■ "A healthy person is simply one who has been inadequately investigated by a teaching hospital." (Draper et al. 1977)

Practice point

Now turn back to the tick exercise on page 43.

If you ticked **1, 9** and **16** you probably think of health in terms of physical fitness, the most obvious component of health. Numbers **5, 7** and **11** may be linked to physical health, but they suggest a notion that being healthy is about not being ill. If you ticked **2** and **10**, then social well-being is important to you. A concern for positive mental health is indicated by you ticking **6, 8** and **12**, whilst numbers **4** and **5** show that emotional health (recognizing and dealing appropriately with emotions as well as coping with stress) is important. The spiritual component of health, which for some people may be concerned with achieving inner peace, for others religious beliefs, is indicated by ticking number **13**.

Think about
What do you think
"being healthy" may
mean to the following
people?

- Someone who is mentally handicapped.
- Someone who has a permanent physical disability such as deafness or paralysis.
- Someone who has an illness or infection for which there is currently no known cure, such as arthritis, HIV or schizophrenia.
- Someone who lives below the poverty line.

You may feel that dividing health into these different components is artificial. Be that as it may, it helps to show how complicated it is to reach an agreed understanding of health. This agreed understanding is especially important for you as a health care worker, dealing with people whose health may be impaired in a variety of ways.

It is vital, when working with people as a health educator, that you find some common ground. *"Start from where they are"* is the basis of **successful communication**.

The word "health" stems from Old English *haelth*, meaning "whole". *An holistic view of health* includes all the components already mentioned, all of which depend to a greater or lesser extent on each other. However, if it is possible for a person to be not totally physically fit, and yet be healthy, could this be true for the other components? It is to be hoped so, for if health is complete well-being, then few of us would ever achieve it!

What affects health?

We live in an unequal society. Inequalities of status, power, employment, housing conditions and many other factors all take their toll on the health of individuals and communities.

The relationship between social conditions and health was noted in 1845 by Engels in *The Conditions of the Working Classes in England*. Engels described the extremes of wealth and poverty and their effects on health.

Personal health is one of the most telling indicators of the degree of in-equality in the UK. Although the health status of the population *as a whole* has steadily improved over the past 200 years, the gap between social classes still exists. Harrison (1983) writes:

Think about
Think about someone
you are caring for. How
would you establish
how that individual
perceives health? What
might this mean for you
as a carer?

❝*Comparing our lowest social group with our highest, we find that unskilled manual workers have three times the rate of limiting long-standing illness as professional and managerial types; four times the rate of mental illness; six times the rate of accidents at work; double the incidence of deafness; three times the*

Think about

Think about the clients you care for or people within your own community. Do some have a better chance of being healthy than others?

incidence of total tooth loss; infant mortality two and a half times as high and still birth rates twice as high. This is inequality incised into the very flesh of the poor. And where the need is greatest the provision is generally the poorest

Some of this is due to social prejudice against specific groups of people, which keeps them living at or below the poverty line. Single parents, elderly people and ethnic minority groups may find themselves confined to a social structure that is so narrow that their choices and their ability to change their circumstances are curtailed.

An issue worthy of comment is whether or not it is possible to separate external influences on health between the **environment**, about which the person can do little, and **lifestyle**, about which the person can make choices. One argument says that personal choices are dictated by environmental factors, such as peer-group pressure to experiment with cigarettes or other drugs, or the availability and cost of "healthy food". On the other hand, some people may feel that smoking is their only pleasure in an otherwise dismal existence. Equally, people who live in a high-rise flat may worry more about their children's physical safety than about low-fat diets.

Practice point
Factors which affect my health

Try this exercise to clarify the factors which affect *your* health. Study the list and arrange the factors into "yes", "no" and "maybe" boxes.

A well-balanced diet	Interesting work
Air pollution	Family
Restful sleep	Where I live
Regular exercise	Stress
Money	Environment
Friends	Noise
Mental stimulation	Love

Feel free to add to this list of factors.

The health of communities

Very few people exist in total isolation. People and their surroundings or community have effects on each other. Communities can be very local to the person (family, street, village, work, college) or may be much larger (town, country, continent, or world). Wilson's definition of health (". . . there is no health for Britain without Bangladesh") asserts that we are all part of the world community.

"Health for all"

In 1978, in the Declaration of Alma Ata (the venue of an international conference), the World Health Organization issued a challenge to the countries of the world to attain health for all by the year 2000. This declaration, to which the UK is a signatory, is based on the belief that health is one of the most important

Think about

How do you think the selection into the boxes would differ for a friend, a partner, a parent, or for one of your clients?

products that any country can create and one of the most important resources required for the creation of any other kind of wealth. The declaration recognized that the successful pursuit of its aim called for fundamental changes in most countries, together with an increased commitment by governments, health service managers, health professionals and researchers as well as those not directly involved in health care.

"Health for All" is not a single finite goal; it involves continuous action by many different agencies and organizations within each country.

The European region of WHO has developed a common health policy for all European countries. The three main elements are:

- the promotion and facilitation of **healthy lifestyles** (aimed at more than individual behaviour change, it requires the establishment of an environment which provides the requirements of healthy living)
- the implementation of measures for the **prevention of disease**
- the provision of **health care** which meets the medical, psychological and social needs of those who need them most in a form which is acceptable to them.

In 1985, the European office of WHO defined 38 targets. It is for each country to interpret these in the context of its own needs and capabilities. The **prerequisites for health** were identified as:

- peace
- social justice
- wholesome food
- safe water
- decent housing
- education
- secure employment

Other European goals were:

- *Addition of years to life* – the prevention of premature death from diseases such as coronary heart disease, stroke, certain cancers, and accidents.
- *Addition of health to life* – the prevention of disease and disability through immunization programmes and antenatal screening.
- *Promotion of healthy behaviour*, and discouraging behaviour which is harmful to self and others.
- *Adoption of policies* to allow the healthy choice to be the easiest choice (e.g. smoking and alcohol policies, greater availability of healthy food).
- *Creation of healthy environments*, such as good housing, clean water, sanitation and Health and Safety at work.
- *Development of appropriate health services.*

"The health of the nation"

In 1992, the UK government published a White Paper entitled *The Health of the Nation: a strategy for health in England*. This emphasizes a commitment to the

Think about
How many of these prerequisites are within an individual's control?

pursuit of "health" in its widest sense, both within government and beyond. It states that, although there is much that the government and the NHS need to do, the objectives and targets cannot be delivered by them alone – identifying the contributions other organizations and agencies can make is essential if the strategy is to succeed. The overall goal of the strategy is to secure continuing improvement in the general health of the population, by "adding years to life and life to years". The strategy emphasizes disease prevention and health promotion as ways in which even greater improvements in health can be secured. The five key areas selected for action are:

- coronary heart disease
- cancers
- mental illness
- HIV/AIDS and sexual health
- accidents.

The White Paper acknowledges the important contribution of the European "Health for All" approach in the formulation of a strategy for health. Success will come through:

- *Public policies* – considering the broad aspects of health when developing policies.
- *Healthy surroundings* – active promotion of physical environments which are conducive to health.
- *Healthy lifestyles* – enabling families and individuals to act on increased knowledge of health.
- *High-quality health services* – identifying and meeting health needs of local populations and securing the balance between health promotion, disease prevention, treatment, care and rehabilitation.

The White Paper encourages active partnerships ("**healthy alliances**") between the many organizations and individuals who can come together to help improve health. Action on a whole variety of fronts will include work in "settings" such as healthy cities, healthy schools, healthy hospitals, with specific action on general health promotion in the workplace and in the environment at large.

Practice point
Make a list of all the things that are happening where you work which could help with the Health of the Nation strategy. Now make a list of new initiatives which you would put in place.

Health promotion and health education

Health promotion is any planned measure which leads to health or prevents disease, disability and premature death. Health promotion has two major components: healthy public policy and health education.

Healthy public policy includes a wide range of measures such as legislation, environmental modification, and various fiscal and economic interventions designed to make healthier choices easier. This applies not only at international and national levels, but also regionally, locally and within organizations such as hospitals, schools and colleges. It is here that "healthy alliances" can play their part.

Health education is the process by which people gain the necessary understanding to make informed choices about health. It includes:

- the process of acquiring health knowledge
- the exploration of attitudes, values and beliefs concerning health
- the acquisition of health, life and social skills needed to facilitate genuine empowered choice.

As a support worker you have the opportunity to contribute to the health of your clients. By being aware of what your clients value and the lifestyle to which they aspire, you can enable them to make *choices* to enhance their well-being. You are in a position to advise on health issues and protect your clients from all forms of discriminatory practice.

To be able to do this you need to know what resources and agencies are available to them and how they might access them. The information you give to clients must be factual and not influenced by your own beliefs and values.

> **Practice point**
> Find out about the organizations and agencies that are available in your own community or area. (Examples are: Health Promotion Unit; Help the Aged; Spastics Society.)

Think about

When contributing to health education it is worth remembering how much is learned from a role model. Think about how you would feel if you were given advice about your diet from a dietitian who was very overweight. How would you feel being advised on the dangers of smoking from a nurse who smokes?

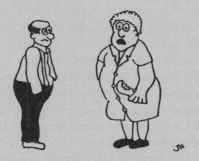

I'M CONCERNED ABOUT YOUR WEIGHT MR SMITH, AND AS A DIETICIAN I NEED TO POINT OUT THE HEALTH RISKS.

Few people working within a care environment would claim to be perfect examples of healthy living, but they do have a responsibility to consider their own health, ways in which it could be improved, and ways in which they could contribute to a healthier environment. Care workers teach by example.

Personal experience can be turned to good advantage. For example, if the dietitian has a constant struggle to control his or her own weight, that experience can be used to develop a greater understanding of clients' difficulties.

Prevention

There is often the mistaken belief that health education is concerned solely with preventing disease and ill-health. The framework of **primary**, **secondary** and **tertiary prevention** and associated health education is a useful one.

Primary prevention

Prevention must always be better than cure. Primary prevention aims to prevent ill-health arising in the first place and is directed at healthy people. Most health education for children and young people falls into this category – dealing with hygiene, contraception, nutrition, and social skills and personal relationships, aiming to build up a positive sense of self-worth. It is also concerned with accident prevention, including campaigning for safer roads and vehicles, as well as educating individuals about safe practices. Primary prevention is concerned not merely with helping to prevent illness, but with positively improving the quality of health and thus the quality of life.

> ### Point to remember
> Your role as a support worker affords you the privileged position of being able to advise and guide individuals, families and the community to behave in ways which are most likely to promote health.

Secondary prevention

This is concerned with action taken *after* the onset of symptoms once a person falls ill. It may be possible to prevent ill-health moving to a chronic or irreversible stage, and restore people to their former state of health.

Restoring health may involve clients in changing their behaviour (such as stopping smoking), following advice and learning about self-care or self-help. Someone who is overweight or who has maturity-onset diabetes will, for example, have to learn how to adjust eating habits to avoid a deterioration in health.

Medications and treatments can be used for specific illnesses, but restoration to a full and useful life can sometimes be achieved only when the entire care team is involved in enabling the client to take control of their health, and changing living practices to reduce self-harm. You will have opportunities to discuss health problems with your clients during your daily contacts with them.

Clients can make decisions regarding their health only if they are provided with all the necessary information from which to draw conclusions. Giving up old, familiar ways of doing things and changing values and ways of thinking can be uncomfortable. Break down the information you give into small pieces – in this way the client may be more willing to be committed to change.

Liaison with health professionals is necessary to ensure that your clients are provided with relevant and up-to-date information.

When trying to help people change their lifestyle you must take into account the danger of forcing your own values upon them, and possibly creating feelings of guilt and anger because the individual cannot comply. Neither can you assume that all people have a genuine ability to choose "healthy" lifestyles, because economic and social factors may have an influence on their freedom of choice.

Point to remember
Good communication skills, and sensitivity to the social, economic, racial and cultural circumstances of clients, are essential when advising or teaching them about healthy options.

Finally, you must always remember to respect the right of individuals to ignore advice on health.

Tertiary prevention

When ill-health has not been or could not be prevented, and someone cannot be restored completely to health, tertiary prevention is concerned with making the most of the remaining potential for healthy living. The aim is to avoid unnecessary hardship restrictions and complications associated with long-term illness, disability or handicap.

Many of your clients will be in this group. Some may have a learning disability or chronic mental illness, whilst others will be terminally ill from a physical condition. Whatever the condition, there are likely to be financial, social, psychological or physical problems which can often be fully resolved. Rehabilitation programmes contain a considerable amount of tertiary health education. Section IV of this book discusses rehabilitation in more detail.

As a support worker, you are vital to the success of tertiary prevention; you will be at the very centre of the lives of your clients, and involved with their families and friends. The opportunities are there for you to ensure that your clients and their families have access to all the people and information they need for their comfort and – frequently – their independence.

Points to remember

- Health is very much a relative concept. It depends not only on the perception of individuals but is also influenced by society and culture.
- Over time, knowledge, experience and social values have affected our approach to health; but as society and technology develops, threats to our health will continue to arise.
- The WHO plays a major part at an international level in directing and coordinating strategies for the promotion and protection of health.
- As a support worker, your role is to work in *partnership* with clients to help them have as much control as possible over their own health. This partnership involves accepting people for what they are, and means that you should:
  - Recognize that people's knowledge and beliefs emerge from their life experiences.

- Understand your own knowledge, beliefs, values and standards.
- Recognize that you and the people you work with may differ in your knowledge, beliefs, values and standards.

Project suggestions

Undertaking project work is an interesting way of learning about a particular topic. Here are some suggestions for a project on health.

- Within your own working area, investigate the potential opportunities for health education and health promotion.
- In your local community, find out what local initiatives for health are being set up and how these might affect you and your clients.
- In how many ways can health issues and messages be communicated to the public?

Further reading

Aggleton (1990), Health (Routledge). Provides a clear and comprehensive introduction to the sociology of health and illness.

Black et al. (1984), Health and Disease – A Reader (Open University). Draws on interdisciplinary research on health in biology, medicine, history and social sciences. Examines the way in which health and disease are defined and the systems that have been developed for coping with them.

Ewles and Simnett (1989), Promoting Health – A Practical Guide (Scutari Press). A day-to-day reference book for most aspects of health education/promotion.

Seedhouse (1986), Health – The Foundations of Achievement (John Wiley). Provides an analysis of and compares a number of different ways of defining health in positive terms.

REFERENCES

Brent Community Health Council (1985). Annual Report, Brent.

Draper, P. et al. (1977) Health and Wealth. *Royal Society of Health Journal*, 97, 121–127.

Harrison, P. (1983). Inside the Inner City – Life Under the Cutting Edge (Harmondsworth: Penguin).

Illych, I. (1976). Limits to Medicine (London, Boyars).

Wilson, M. (1976). Health is for People. (Dartington: Longman and Todd).

Mental health

6

Damon Britton

For many years, mental health problems have been isolated in their recognition and acceptance. This is not because of their scarcity – far from it. Rather it is due to the stigma they have carried and to some extent still carry. This chapter is designed to be of benefit to health care workers who come into contact with clients in any capacity, not just those working specifically in the mental health field.

Although this chapter focuses on mental health, as a health care worker you will encounter clients with a variety of psychological problems in a variety of care settings. The promotion of their mental well-being is consequently of paramount importance.

When caring for people who have mental health problems, or difficulties maintaining their psychological well-being, the carer should always take into account the individuality and complexities of human nature.

The key issues of this chapter are:
- The self, and elements that may interfere with caring
- Key aspects of communication skills
- Awareness of how to implement these skills when faced with aggression
- Insight into people at risk and what "at risk" means
- The Mental Health Act 1983 and the carer's role in its implementation
- Helping to maintain and promote mental health.

Looking at self-awareness

As a support worker you will not be immune from prejudice, or negative and sometimes harmful attitudes and conceptions towards certain groups of people, such as those with a mental illness or a learning or physical disability. You may also be against the use of certain treatments such as abortion and electroplexy (ECT).

To be able to help your clients effectively you must be able to *identify* these

This chapter links to Unit O and endorsement units Z1, Z2, Z3, Z4, Z8, U4.

attitudes and beliefs within yourself, and actively prevent them from interfering with your interactions with clients.

Example

John is an intensive-care nurse who feels a great frustration when caring for a patient who has attempted suicide and therefore apparently "wants to die". He feels his skills and abilities would be better served on the patients who require intensive nursing and who desperately "want to live". These frustrations and beliefs have to be allayed for John to be able to care for his suicidal patient in an unconditional and empathetic way and to give the patient the equality of care deserved.

Think about

Read the statements below and decide, on a scale of 1 to 5, how much you agree or disagree (1 = do not agree, 5 = strongly agree).

"Everyone who suffers from a mental illness is aggressive."

"Homosexuality is an illness."

"All hippies take drugs."

"Black people are better athletes than white people."

"Asians prefer to be cared for by Asians."

Add your scores together. If you score above 5 and have rated yourself honestly, you have identified an element of prejudice within you.

Think about

Recall a time when you were trying to have a conversation with a friend or family member and you knew they were not listening. How did you know they were not listening? (Think of body positioning, eye contact, response or lack of it. . . .) Did this make you feel ignored, worthless, devalued, angry, frustrated, uninteresting, upset?

If one of your clients is attempting to tell you something vitally important and you are giving them the impression that you are not listening, that client will have very similar feelings to the ones you have experienced.

Having an element of prejudice does not prevent you from being an effective carer. Identifying the prejudice is the beginning of awareness of your feelings towards other people. You have the chance to look at how you can be less prejudiced and consequently be able to listen objectively to your clients with an accurate understanding.

Communication skills during interactions

Being able to **listen** and **communicate effectively** are key skills when it comes to helping a client with mental health problems. You may be thinking "*Of course I listen when somebody is talking to me*"; but are you being totally honest? How do you make it known to the other person that you are listening to what they have to say?

Point to remember

Listening is not just a passive process of sitting back, letting your ears do the work. It is an active experience of reading verbal and non-verbal messages in the act of communicating.

A guide to the principles of showing active listening as described by Gerard Egan (1982) can be summed up in the mnemonic **soler**:

s Face your client *squarely*; i.e. adopt a posture that shows you are interested and involved.

o Adopt an *open* posture; crossed arms and legs can be interpreted as a sign of disinterest.

l *Leaning* gently towards your client can show that you are interested.

e Maintain *eye* contact, but do not stare.

r Try to appear *relaxed* during your interactions.

Verbal prompts, too, can be a good sign of active listening. They show the client that you are interested. Prompts such as "uh huh", "yes", "go on", are commonly used.

Thus we communicate on two levels – verbally and non-verbally. **Verbal communication** consists of the things that are spoken and, when taken at face value, transmits factual information accurately and efficiently. **Non-verbal communication** consists of a number of elements, including tone of voice, eye contact, body posture, gestures, touch, and facial expression. It has been estimated (Mehrabain 1972) that 7% of communication is transmitted by words, 38% by vocal cues like tone of voice, and 55% by body cues such as facial expression.

Example

"I'm OK" implies that your client is feeling well. But if it were said whilst the person was sitting with arms folded across his chest, looking at the floor and rocking backwards and forwards, it could have a totally different implication.

When you are actively listening and communicating you need to be aware of everything your client is saying and doing. This is not as hard as it sounds. It is just an extension of what you are doing every day during every interaction with another person. *However, it is also a skill to be able to do this therapeutically and needs to be practised.*

Non-verbal communication

Factors to take into account when understanding non-verbal communication are:

- posture
- facial expressions
- eyes
- touching
- gestures and body movements

Posture can be defined as your total body attitude. It can refer either to the general way in which you behave or to a particular position that is adopted. For example, standing with legs apart and hands on hips indicates an authoritative stance; sitting with legs and arms crossed with head downwards indicates a defensive/isolative position; standing with legs apart, arms raised, and hands clenched indicates an aggressive stance.

The **face** is the most expressive part of the body. **Facial expressions** can indicate any number of moods and emotional responses, such as happiness, sadness, horror, anxiety, fear, puzzlement, indecision, boredom, concentration.

The **eyes** were described by St Augustine as "the windows of the soul". They can reveal any number of emotions and inner feelings. The eyes can be a good guide when it is difficult to read a person's facial expressions.

Touching involves both personal space and action. It is a good way to communicate understanding and empathy, or to offer warmth and reassurance. But be aware that not every client responds positively to touch, and you should feel comfortable with your understanding of your client before using this.

Gestures and body movements are the way the body and limbs are used to convey signals. For example, shoulder shrugging may mean "I don't understand". A closed hand with thumb in the air may mean "I'm OK". Hands over both ears may mean "I don't want to listen to you any more". It must be stressed that *although many of these gestures and body movements have a universal meaning you must take into account your client's culture and society*, to avoid any possible misinterpretation. Some simple gestures are considered obscene in some cultures.

Effective communication skills are important when you are looking after somebody who is in need of help. Although these skills come naturally to a large extent, you do need to be aware and need to practise and develop the skills if they are to be of therapeutic value.

Dealing with aggressive incidents

When interacting with your clients, within a relaxed and friendly environment, it is quite common to underestimate the importance of being aware of how you are communicating or appearing. However, if you are faced by a client who is extremely upset or angry, the value of this awareness is more apparent.

Violence within health care is thankfully very rare, but as a support worker you may at some point be faced with a client or relative presenting aggressive behaviour.

Aggression in itself is not always a negative response to a situation. Indeed, it is needed in all of us to gain independence and achievement in life, and to assert our own individuality. However, on occasions aggression is associated with a sudden discharge of emotions in response to fear or frustration. This is **negative aggression**. It can be subdivided into four types:

- *assaultive* – aimed at people
- *destructive* – directed at the environment
- *passive* – a withdrawal from interactions/society
- *internalized* – directed against the self.

Proactive intervention

Clients have needs. If these are not being met then they will experience feelings of frustration, unworthiness, devaluation or anger. If left unresolved these feelings may then "boil over" into an aggressive response. It is your responsibility as a

Think about

Can you remember the last time you had to sit and wait for what seemed an age to be served in a restaurant? How did you feel (frustrated, unimportant, devalued, angry)? It is quite likely that if you were left for any length of time these feelings would begin to manifest themselves as aggressive behaviour.

Try to put yourself in the place of a client who, on seeking attention or time from you as a support worker, is told "I'm very busy at the moment, I won't be long", or "Can't it wait?"

support worker to be **proactive** in the prevention of the build-up of these emotions.

This means being aware of your client's needs, environment, idiosyncrasies, anxieties and problems. Proactive intervention involves helping clients to find ways of avoiding situations which may lead to aggressive outbursts, or ways of coping with their emotions before resorting to aggression.

> **Point to remember**
> If you were being **reactive** you would wait until your client was being aggressive before attempting to resolve the situation. **By this time it may be too late!**

Proactive intervention is therefore a more effective way of caring and will lead to a more positive response. If you are using your effective communication skills to build up a trusting and therapeutic relationship with your client, then most aggressive situations will be prevented. This is healthier for both you and your client.

The fight/flight phenomenon

Occasionally, no matter how skilled your proactive interventions may be, you will be faced with a client who is displaying aggressive behaviour. It is important to have an understanding of what the client is experiencing both physically and psychologically.

When a client is displaying aggressive behaviour, his mind is preparing him to deal with what it perceives to be an emergency situation. He can either fight (i.e. face the situation) or take flight (run from the situation). This is called the "**fight/flight reaction**". The client experiences both a *physical* and a *psychological* response to the situation.

Physically he will have:

- increased heart rate and palpitations
- increased blood pressure
- increased respiration rate (hyperventilation)
- pupil dilation
- increased digestion rate ("butterflies in tummy")
- agitation and restlessness
- tremor
- either flushed expression or pallor.

Psychologically he will have:

- hyperalertness
- increased speed of thought processes
- hypersensitivity
- thought blocks
- feelings of fear or loss of control.

> **Think about**
> Do you recognize any of these feelings from your wait in the restaurant?

Reactive intervention

Reactive intervention may be necessary in an attempt to calm the situation and prevent it from turning to violence.

> **Point to remember**
>
> When attempting to help a client who is demonstrating assaultive or destructive aggression, before intervening you must ask yourself three questions:
>
> ■ Am I safe?
> ■ Is the client safe?
> ■ Are people in the vicinity safe?
>
> If you answer no to any of the three questions, GET SUPPORT. This does not mean fetching the front row of the local rugby team, which would only antagonize the situation. Rather, ensure that appropriate colleagues are discreetly close by, to remove onlookers from the area and to help you if violence is a possibility.

Then, when it is safe to do so, approach the client calmly. Keep control of your own feelings – you too will be experiencing the fight/flight reaction.

■ Use an open non-threatening posture and manner.
■ Listen to what the patient is saying (and show it).
■ Maintain eye contact, but don't stare.

Talk to the client, and use **relaxation techniques** to help the client to regain control of his body's response. Ask your client to take slow deep breaths – this will alleviate hyperventilation, reduce the heart rate and palpitations. Offer the opportunity to sit down and talk through the problem. *Absorb any verbal abuse –* do not respond or react.

Use your knowledge and understanding of your client. If humour helps, use it. If distraction works, use it. If giving space and time works, use it. If you know your client well, then non-threatening touch is useful; but be aware that not everybody likes to be touched and always be aware of personal space.

Finally, **maintain dignity** by guiding your client to a private area of the ward when it is safe to do so. *Always use your communication skills throughout.*

After the incident

Once an incident of aggressive outbursts has been resolved, it is important that you are given time to regain control of your own feelings and physiological responses. You can do this by discussing the incident with your colleagues, asking for feedback on how the situation was handled, and analysing any possible ways the situation could have been prevented (i.e. at what point did proactive interventions fail?). Have a cup of tea!

It is equally important to give your client the opportunity to discuss the incident. The client may feel rejected, guilty or frightened of rebuff because of the outburst. By talking through the incident with the client, you are helping to prevent any build-up of "bad feelings" and maintaining the therapeutic relationship. Your care continues by looking at possible ways of preventing similar outbursts.

People at risk

The term "at risk" is usually attributed to a client when his or her ability to keep safe from harm has in some way been impaired. For clients with a mental health problem, "at risk" may come under the following categories:

- suicide
- parasuicide (the deliberate act of self harm which does not have a fatal outcome (Hawton and Catalan 1982)
- accidental injury
- neglect.

Care for clients who fit into the first three categories is initially based around crisis (or reactive) interventions, which rely wholeheartedly on communication skills and the development of a therapeutic relationship. The main aim is to prevent injury or further attempts at suicide, until the client is able to take responsibility once more. In the case of parasuicide this involves great risk-taking and may mean at times giving clients back responsibility before they have ceased harming themselves, whilst at the same time helping them to develop alternative healthier strategies for coping.

When a client is deemed "at risk", an intervention commonly used is sometimes referred to as **Special Nursing Observations**. These vary slightly from hospital to hospital, but they usually have the core ingredients of three levels.

Level 1

The client is to be within touching distance of the nurse/carer at all times. The only exception may be when the client is in the toilet, where the nurse/carer must be positioned immediately outside the door and the door must not be locked. The client may not leave the ward unless to attend essential or urgent appointments and must then be under nurse escort, usually a minimum of two.

Level 2

The same as level 1 except that the client must be in vision at all times rather than within touching distance.

Level 3

The client's whereabouts must be known at all times by an allocated nurse or carer, and a visual check must be made on the client at intervals specified in the Nursing Care Plan. The client may not leave the ward unless with a nurse escort.

Think about

Think about levels 1 and 2 of the Special Nursing Observations. How would you feel if you had somebody watching you all the time and they were actively trying to prevent you from doing something you really wanted to do? Would you feel angry, frustrated, betrayed, embarrassed, suspicious, isolated, imprisoned?

Carrying out these observations requires a lot of skill and patience and at times may be very stressful to both the client and carer. The carer must not be viewed as standing on "guard duty" as this means the message being given to the client is one of punishment rather than caring. The situation should rather be viewed as an excellent opportunity to begin or continue the process of establishing rapport and building a therapeutic relationship. Ultimately this shows your client that somebody is interested in their well-being and safety.

Always be aware, however, that if a person wishes to' die and you are preventing this, in all likelihood that person is observing you as closely as you are observing him or her. It is therefore imperative that the client's behaviour, thought content, interaction levels and significant conversation content are recorded in the nursing notes/observation care plan, as these are all important indicators of intent.

Dealing with neglect

Neglect usually emanates from the illnesses of depression, mania, psychosis or substance abuse. However, it should be remembered that it is also one way of committing suicide, so note should always be taken that as your client's well-being improves so may his or her motivation to find alternative ways to commit suicide.

The nursing care is again usually crisis intervention, but you are mainly aiming at the common components of daily living such as eating, drinking, personal hygiene and elimination. In extreme circumstances you need to take responsibility in helping clients to maintain these to the standard at which they functioned before illness.

You must remember always that it is your role to promote independence. The client must be encouraged to carry out as many of these functions as seems reasonable, giving back total responsibility as soon as possible.

Approaching discharge

When a client has regained his or her psychological well-being and is about to be discharged, there will be anxiety at the thought of returning to the environment where the original problems were experienced. You should continue to be proactive by helping your client to identify support services available on discharge, and by discussing any possible need for their involvement. Possibilities are community psychiatric nurse (CPN) or GP involvement for continued support; the Samaritans for a contact if problems again begin to get out of control; even friends or the next-door neighbour as someone to listen and share their worries.

Caring within the Mental Health Act 1983

People who are deemed "at risk" are sometimes too ill to realize that they need specialist care or inpatient treatment. It is occasionally necessary to admit or treat someone in hospital against their will or without their consent.

A law for the protection of people suffering from mental health problems has

Practice point
Are you aware of the support services available to your clients? Make a list of:
► the phone number of your local Samaritans
► any counselling services available
► any other support services appropriate to your clients' care, either professional or voluntary.

been in existence in one form or another since the opening of Bethlam hospital in 1274. Until 1954 the law had been used primarily to "protect the public from the insane". However, since 1954 the outlook on mental health problems has altered, and the Mental Health Act 1983 is used primarily for the protection of the client who is deemed to be a risk to themselves or others.

The Act itself is a lengthy official document. It is divided into sections covering various aspects of detaining, assessing, or treating a person against his or her will and is available to any one who wishes further information. As a support worker in hospital or community settings, you are most likely to come across the sections listed below:

Section 2   Admission for Assessment (up to 28 days)
Section 3   Admission for treatment (up to 6 months initially)
Section 5(2)   Detention for up to 72 hours
Section 5(4)   Detention for up to 6 hours

Section 2 – admission for assessment

This is admission to or detention in hospital for a client suffering from mental health problems to a degree that warrants assessment (or assessment followed by treatment) for at least a limited period. The client is detained in the interests of his or her health and safety, or for the protection of others.

Detention is for up to 28 days, and an application for detention must be made by the client's nearest relative or an approved social worker. This application must be supported by the written recommendation of two medical practitioners, one of whom should be approved as having special experience in the treatment and diagnosis of mental illness, and the other should have previous knowledge of the client.

Section 3 – admission for treatment

This is admission to or detention in hospital for a client suffering from mental health problems to such a degree that medical treatment in hospital is necessary. The client is detained for his or her own health and safety, or for the protection of others. The application and medical recommendations are as in Section 2.

The section runs for a maximum of 6 months but can be renewed if treatment is deemed necessary after this time limit has expired.

Treatment against the client's wishes can only be carried out for a maximum of 3 months. If it is to continue for longer, a second opinion must be sought from the Mental Health Act Commission.

Section 5(2) – detention for up to 72 hours

This is for clients already in hospital who, although wishing to leave, are not allowed to leave in the interests of their health and safety, and that of others who may be put at risk.

The recommendation for detention can be made by a doctor who feels that an application for longer admission or treatment needs to be made but where the client is unwilling to stay in hospital while this is achieved.

Section 5(4) – detention for up to 6 hours

This section is similar to section 5(2). A registered mental nurse in charge may detain the client, for a maximum of 6 hours. If the 6 hours elapse and the doctor has not arrived, the section is *not* renewable and the client must be allowed to leave.

Keeping the client informed

It is very unlikely that you as a support worker will be involved in the intricate workings of the Act. However, you will have a very important role in *informing* clients of their rights under the Act, acting as their supporter at all times, and bringing to the attention of the relevant person in charge any discrepancies in care or detention.

Every hospital has a duty to supply information to detained clients and their relatives, and this usually comes in the form of a leaflet. Sitting down with your client and reading through the leaflet together may seem pointless, or even condescending, but it demonstrates concern for your client's well-being. It ensures that the client has a full understanding of his or her rights, particularly where the detention is forced.

Think about it from the client's perspective. The nurses and support workers he (or she) has come to like and trust have suddenly become the people who are implementing a law which means he has to be detained even though he has not committed any crime. He may feel let down, cheated or even betrayed. He needs to understand that he has not been rejected and that your ultimate aim is to help him regain his mental health and eventual return home.

By helping him understand his rights under the Act, you are aiding in his empowerment to appeal against his detention. By giving the information he needs to obtain help in that appeal, you are showing him that he has not been rejected and that you are maintaining the therapeutic relationship. You maintain your role of supporter by speaking on behalf of your client, not only in relation to the Mental Health Act, but also in all aspects of care and treatment which may compromise his rights. Your client has someone to turn to for explanation of his care, or of words and terms he does not understand. Being your client's supporter is, however, extremely difficult at times, especially if there is a conflict of interests.

Client appeals

A client who has been detained under section 2 of the Act may appeal to the Mental Health Review Tribunal (MHRT) within 14 days of detention. Under section 3 of the Act the appeal may be at any time within the 6 months. Alternatively the person can appeal to the hospital managers, where there is no time limit. Both the MHRT and managers have the power to rescind the order, and both use the same process of interviewing the client, doctor, named nurse and social worker informally to reach this decision. The client has no rights of appeal under sections 5(2) and 5(4).

The client may elect to have another person present at the interview to provide some moral support. That other person may be their solicitor, a relative or yourself.

Think about

You are caring for a client who is extremely poorly from alcohol abuse. However, he has no insight into this and says he feels OK. You discover that he has managed to secrete a bottle of spirits into his locker. You are aware that the client has a right to ignore good health advice, but equally you realize that your client needs to adhere to his treatment. By reporting this to your senior, are you ignoring the rights of the client? You may wish to discuss this idea with colleagues.

It is not unusual for the support worker to be asked to help the client to write a letter to the managers or MHRT for an appeal. Again, by doing this you are showing your client that you care and value his or her rights as an individual.

If your client feels unfairly treated under the Mental Health Act, he or she can write to the Mental Health Act Commission. The Commission was set up to ensure that clients' rights are not compromised by the Act, and all complaints are investigated.

Maintaining mental health

The Mental Health Act is implemented only in cases of extreme need, and more often than not as the final part of crisis intervention. It is, however, part of your role as a health care worker to promote the maintenance of mental health and thereby be proactive in the care not only of your clients and their carers but also of yourself.

This is also consistent with the process of returning to your clients the responsibility for their own well-being and health, to the point that the only help they will continue to need is support.

One definition of mental health is as follows:

Mental health is psychological well-being or adequate adjustment, particularly where the adjustment conforms to the community accepted standards of human relations.

Some of these characteristics are (Cambell and Hinsie 1989):

- reasonable independence
- self-reliance
- self-direction
- ability to do a job
- ability to take responsibility and make needed efforts
- reliability
- persistence
- ability to get along with others
- cooperation
- ability to give and take
- ability to work under authority, rules and difficulties
- ability to show friendliness and love
- tolerance of others and of frustrations
- ability to contribute
- sense of humour
- devotion beyond self
- ability to find recreation/hobbies

In helping your clients to maintain these characteristics you adopt the role of **health educator**. As a health educator you must work with your clients to help them identify the factors which are potentially stressful. Even when the problems have been identified there is no guarantee of an instant solution, but being able to recognize the potential problems is helpful in itself. The client can then be given the opportunity to learn **coping skills**.

Stress is not *altogether* unhealthy, in that it can provide the stimulus to keep you positive and well-motivated, and strengthen existing coping mechanisms. An absence of stress (which may sound wonderful) would imply a very boring life.

Think about
How would your life be affected if you broke your leg? Consider these aspects: employment, finances, relationships, independence, security; role as mother/father, partner, provider.

Table 6.1   Scoring the effects of life changes

Life events	LCUs
Death of spouse	100
Divorce	73
Marital separation	65
Jail term	63
Death of close family member	63
Personal injury or illness	53
Marriage	50
Pregnancy	40
Moving house	20
Change in eating habits	15
Holiday	13

Think about
Imagine your client following your advice to take up mountaineering, only to realize half-way up a rock face that he is afraid of heights. That is not an ideal way to relieve stress! It is important for clients to be given realistic options which will allow them to select coping strategies to suit their abilities and lifestyles.

In present-day society stress and anxiety are unavoidable, and they have been identified as major factors in influencing mental health. Therefore, by identifying the major **stressors** and helping your clients to learn healthy ways of coping with them you will play an important role in the maintenance of mental health. As described in Chapter 5, you should encourage clients to look at their lives *holistically*. This means helping them to look at the physical, psychological, social, sexual and spiritual aspects and identifying any areas which may be problematic. If one area is not functioning effectively this can have a negative effect on other areas, resulting in stress.

A team at the University of Washington (Holmes and Rahe 1967) developed a scale for measuring the seriousness of life events. The more stressful the event, the higher the "life-change units" or LCUs (see Table 6.1). If an individual's life-change units total over 300, it is believed that he or she runs a high risk of suffering a major illness within the following two years.

You will have your own coping mechanisms for dealing with stress, both healthy (playing sport, relaxation, hobbies) and unhealthy (having an alcoholic drink after a hard day at work, shouting at your partner). These will be idiosyncratic to yourself, so it is of no use saying to your client "When you leave hospital you should take up mountaineering – it works wonders for me." Your clients need to identify for themselves what will be beneficial and helpful.

As a health care worker and someone your client looks to for help, you need to be aware of different options and be supportive when exploring possibilities. Some options may be:

Think about
Think about other possible coping strategies, but always be receptive to suggestions made by your client.

- relaxation techniques
- anxiety and stress management techniques
- seeking support from others
- distraction techniques
- creating personal space.

In your role as an educator, do not be blinkered into thinking only about your client. Always remember that others in contact with the client – spouse, partner, neighbours, friends – will also be affected by your client's problems and may also benefit from your help and guidance.

Drug treatment compliance

Health education is not restricted to developing coping strategies. Clients with certain forms of mental health problems (e.g. depression, schizophrenia, manic/depressive psychosis) may be undergoing long-term drug treatment. It is imperative that clients understand the importance of continuing with the prescribed medication, and be warned of the possibilities of relapse if medication is stopped without support from a relevant professional.

Frequently a client will stabilize well on medication, only to cease taking it because he or she cannot see the reason to continue, often with tragic results. With the correct information and help this should not occur and the client's health will be maintained.

Have you ever been prescribed a course of antibiotics? You will probably have found that after the first couple of days the symptoms of your illness eased dramatically. It is at this point that a great many people stop taking their antibiotic medication without realizing that they should continue for the full course prescribed, as the infection itself has not been eradicated. *The same principal applies to medication linked with mental health.* Although it is not generally prescribed for a specific length of time, your client should not cease taking it because the symptoms have cleared or eased.

Points to remember

- Mental health problems can occur in anyone, anywhere and at any time. Such problems are most likely to occur at times of crisis, in particular during periods of physical ill-health in the individual or ill-health in a partner, friend or loved one. Divorce, unemployment or bereavement may also trigger a mental health problem.
- Disruption to the normal lifestyle, and loss of control of any activity of daily living, can lead to reduced self-esteem. A lack of power to change these circumstances leads to frustration which may manifest itself in aggression, self-harm, withdrawal or other psychological disturbance.
- Your knowledge of the causes and signs of disturbed equilibrium will enable you to instigate interventions to help clients, carers and friends, to regain or maintain their psychological well-being.
- *Don't forget yourself.* Keep looking at your own lifestyle, continue to identify areas of stress in your own life, develop healthy coping strategies and, most of all, keep working to maintain your own mental health. In doing so you will be in a much better position to help the clients who are seeking your care.

Further reading

Collister (1988), Psychiatric Nursing (Edward Arnold). Easy to understand and follow, showing nursing in all areas of mental health.

Ironbar and Hooper (1989), Self Instruction in Mental Health Nursing (Baillière Tindall). A good guide to anybody using the skills involved in mental health nursing.

Rogers (1973), Person to Person—The Problem of Being Human (Souvenir Press).

Egan (1982), The Skilled Helper (Brookes/Cole Publishing, Monterey, California). One of the forerunners of modern counselling and interpersonal relationships. Excellent for identifying and using non-verbal communication skills.

REFERENCES

Cambell, J.R. and Hinsie, L.E. (1989). *Psychiatric Dictionary*, 6th edn, (Oxford University Press).

Egan, G. (1982). *The Skilled Helper: A model for systematic helping and interpersonal relating*, Brookes/Cole Publishing.

Hawton, K. and Catalan, J. (1982). *Attempted Suicide*, Oxford University Press.

Holmes, T. and Rahe, R. (1967). *Journal of Psychosomatic Research*, 11, 213.

Mehrabain, A. (1972). *Non-Verbal Communication*, Aldine Publishing.

Healthy attitudes to ageing

7

Judith Wilson

In the western world the majority of people expect to live beyond "three score years and ten", and over the past 100 years there has been a rise in the proportion of elderly people within the community.

Life expectancy differs in different parts of the world and between the sexes. In Japan, men can expect to live to 75 and women to 81 years, yet in Hungary the life expectancy for men is only 65 and for women 71 years. In the UK the expectancies are 72 for men and 78 for women.

Our society is large and complex but with a certain amount of categorization. This means that groups of people are often "labelled". Chapter 8 describes how a label can have a detrimental effect on the way people are perceived and how they will respond to others. Similarly, elderly people suffer from stereotyped viewpoints. This chapter is about dispelling such views. It promotes a more positive attitude towards people in the later stage of their lives.

If we are to encourage independent living, we must take steps to ensure that the quality of life for the elderly is both promoted and maintained.

The key issues of this chapter are:
- Who are "the elderly"?
- How old is "old"?
- Attitudes to ageing
- Myths associated with ageing
- Ageism
- Abuse

This chapter links with units O, Z1, Z4 and applies to *all* carers wherever they work, not just those involved exclusively with the elderly.

Who are "the elderly"?

When you look around, where you work and in your local community, do you see more elderly men than women, or vice versa? It is quite likely that you will notice more women than men, and there are a number of reasons why this is so. Firstly, men have traditionally worked in more hazardous conditions than women.

Secondly, men have tended to drink more alcohol, smoke more and have a higher incidence of stress-related diseases. Thirdly, there are more men than women in the armed services, and over the last 100 years conflicts throughout the world have claimed the lives of many young men.

Perceptions of old age

The term "old" has no fixed meaning. To a child, it may mean a chronological age of 20. To a teenager, someone of 30 or 40 is already "over the hill" or "past it". To a person of 70, "old" means older than oneself.

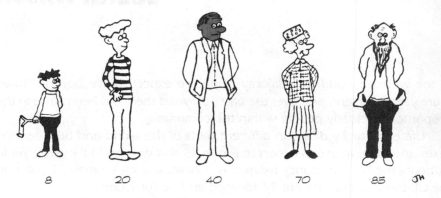

8   20   40   70   85

Think about

Are you looking forward to being old? Your answer will probably be an emphatic NO. Why?

Is it because you have the preconceived notion that being old automatically means infirmity and decrepitude? Is it because advancing years take away all that we have spent years trying to attain, including the zest for life, robust health, total involvement in the world around us and the ability to contribute actively to life?

Ask your family and friends how they perceive "old" and what it means to them.

You might consider growing old in a different light when you have studied the following statistics:

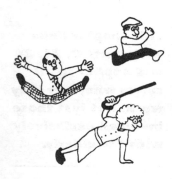

- Eight out of ten people (80%) over the age of 75 have no complaint of restriction of activity on the grounds of poor health.
- Most old people (72% of those over 70) need no help to live at home; and of those who do, 90% are helped by their families.
- Fewer than 4% of those over 65 live in any form of non-domestic (institutional) setting.
- At least 80% of people over 80 have not the slightest evidence of dementia.

These statistics portray a robust, cheerful picture of independence – as opposed to the general **stereotype** of old-age as a time of frailty, helplessness, gradual decline and irreversible disability. Unfortunately, these perceptions are deeply ingrained, more particularly in western society.

Other societies treat their elderly with a great deal of respect and honour, valuing their knowledge and understanding of the world. The Chinese in particular have a notable tradition of bestowing high status upon their older members, the eldest son taking responsibility for the care of his elderly parents. There are many other cultures which pay careful attention to the physical, social and spiritual needs of the elderly within the community.

Think about:
"When an elderly person dies, a library is lost."

How old is "old"?
Old-age can be visualized as a person who has reached a certain number of years, or it can be thought of as a description of a state of life with certain characteristics. Perhaps old-age could be described as having reached a certain stage in life. A person negotiates the First Age of education and childhood, and the Second Age of work and possibly raising a family. There follows the Third Age of active retirement, and the Fourth Age of dependence and eventual death. All of these descriptions are *relative*. As to when a person should be called "old", views have varied – ancient Romans were *senex* at 45 years.

Very few people actually think of themselves as being old and most people do not know what "feeling old" means. They have to remind themselves of the number of years they have lived.

Table 7.1   Age distribution of the UK population (in thousands)

	1901	1931	1951	1971	1981	1991
Male						
65–74	565	1099	1561	1976	2210	2266
75+	219	372	687	628	1091	1349
Female						
60–64	577	1003	1361	1709	1510	1502
65–69	411	792	1183	1511	1497	1509
80–84	94	165	317	546	642	825
All						
65–74	1278	2461	3689	4713	5049	5062
75+	531	957	1777	2594	3120	3748

Source: Office of Population Censuses and Surveys

From a historical point of view, Table 7.1 shows the increase in the numbers of people living to a greater age in the UK.

By the year 2000 the percentages between the bandings will change and there will be:

■ a decrease in the number between 65 and 75
■ a small increase (7%) in those aged 75–85

Practice point
Look around your local community and work area. If you have older relatives, think about their lives and friends. You may wish to ask them about how long their parents and grandparents lived, and how the elderly were perceived in those times.

■ a large increase (29%) in the over-80s, and as much as 34% in the 85+ group.

All this information shows that in the future there are likely to be more people who will need care in some form or another, although not as much as you might have thought. A large proportion of the elderly population lead independent lives.

Retirement

Retirement is one of the major social and emotional changes that will affect all individuals in their later years. It is a major milestone in life and one which describes a change in role and social status.

The retirement age of 65 for men was introduced in the UK in 1886, when the life expectancy was approximately 40 years. Since then life expectancy has increased but not the retirement age.

Retiring from paid employment can have a marked impact on people both financially and socially. Some people may continue to work longer, dependent upon their occupation, and women will often continue to care for their home for much longer. Some people may choose to retire early.

Attitudes to ageing

Individual views of ageing arise from personal experiences with relatives, friends and colleagues and with the society in which we live. The cultural background plays an important role in the development of ideas and opinions, and the media have a strong influence on how the elderly are portrayed. When watching television, note how often the advertisers use "young and beautiful" people to promote their products.

In many societies people are classified as "old" when they reach a particular age and are then treated in a different way – often with the assumption that at that age the person is no longer capable.

Point to remember
As carers we need to be clear about our own values and beliefs regarding the elderly, to ensure that our verbal and non-verbal behaviour does not project negative feelings.

Think about
Think about someone you know who has retired within the past two or three years. What differences has it made to their lifestyle? Has it altered *your* attitude or behaviour toward them?

For some people, caring for the elderly is seen as dull and full of routine – not very exciting. An A&E department or coronary care unit may seem to have more appeal. It is important to remember that things are not all "doom and gloom" when people get old. The skills of the elderly are a much undervalued resource and their need to give often goes unrecognized. In many ways, caring for the elderly is more fulfilling than working in an A&E department because of the opportunities for giving friendship and understanding, and the opportunities for communication and social interaction.

Five myths associated with ageing

Myth 1: Elderly people revert to childhood

An elderly person *never* reverts to childhood. This myth has arisen because some elderly people develop physical problems which result in a reduction of their dexterity, and in some cases an inability to be fully in control of their bodily functions. This does not remove **adult status**.

> **Think about**
> ▶ How do you feel when you are with older adults, grandparents, aunts, uncles?
> ▶ How do you react when someone repeats things over and over again?
> ▶ How do you feel when someone takes a long time to perform a simple activity like putting on an article of clothing?
> ▶ Do you make negative assumptions about an elderly person's capability?

Myth 2: Elderly people have reduced intellect and enjoy childish games

Whilst pathological changes do sometimes occur, as in **dementia**, intelligence level does not change. With increasing age, **memory** for recent events often does diminish but this may have something to do with the fact that the longer you live the more you have to remember! In fact, if a person keeps mentally active and retains an interest in life and living, he or she will be just as intelligent as they ever were. A number of "elderly" people achieve university degrees.

Myth 3: Most older adults are lonely and socially isolated

The older a person becomes the more likely it is that their family and social network will have shrunk. Many, especially those over the age of 75, live on their own. However, this does not necessarily mean they are without social contacts.

Being alone does not mean the same as being lonely. It is a myth that everyone must have constant company. People need personal space and individuals should be able to choose if and when they wish to be alone. The sensitive carer will be able to strike a balance in the provision of **social interaction** and **privacy**.

For some people who have lived on their own, going into a nursing home or residential home, or even going to live with their family, may be a difficult transition to make. Many carers are tempted to say "The company will be good for you", without justification.

Myth 4: The elderly no longer have the same feelings and emotions

It is important for people to express their personality through their outward appearance. Personal dignity and self-respect is a vital component of individuality.

> **Think about**
>
> Consider the following statements:
> - The elderly do not mind wearing communal clothes.
> - They do not mind being stripped naked in front of strangers.
> - They do not mind being taken to the toilet and seen by a stranger.
>
> If you were to be treated in this way by people, what would it tell you about their opinion of you?

Myth 5: The elderly find sexuality and sexual activity distasteful

Sexuality is about individuality and self-perception. Sexual activity may decline with the years and with the non-availability of a partner, but emotional and physical needs remain. It is not "how often" that matters but the quality, and this applies equally to any age group. It seems that we may have very liberal attitudes towards the young but not to the old.

The elderly themselves are reluctant to express their sexual feelings for fear of being seen as depraved or lecherous. Thus, myths about their sexuality are internalized and result in frustration. This frustration often manifests itself in "difficult" behaviour. The belief that sex no longer matters is totally unfounded.

It is sometimes thought that separating the sexes in care settings will avoid problems for both staff and families. Research has shown that where elderly men and women are free to mix in a normal social environment, they are less tense, are better groomed, and retain an interest in social activities. It is the *carers* who have found some difficulty in accepting that sexuality remains a normal part of the human psyche, however old one is.

> **Point to remember**
>
> *These five myths are all too common. Such beliefs colour our relationships with older adults and build barriers to mutual respect and understanding. It is important to be aware of the normal ageing process in an effort to dispel such myths, not only for the carer but for the elderly as well.*

Ageism

The term **ageism** emerged in the USA in the 1960s and has been introduced into our everyday language. It is a label which implies a degree of stereotyping and discrimination towards older people. In a similar way, sexism and racism are discrimination against those of differing sex or race.

Ageism allows the young to see the elderly as being "different". This in turn excuses the young from thinking about things they would rather not consider (e.g. illness, ageing and death). Thus they subtly cease to identify with their elders as human beings.

In modern society where payment for work is important, the elderly are frequently seen as being **unproductive** and not worth while. Society imposes this non-role on people when they reach that "certain age" (whatever that might be).

Ageism thus produces negative attitudes. This viewpoint can be seen in the carer who becomes annoyed when asked to look after an older client, or who displays irritation if the client does not move "fast enough". There is a belief that all old people are rude, difficult and awkward, but can we not honestly say the same of people from all walks of life?

Carers need to learn from older people about how they feel and how they have coped with the changes in their physical, social and emotional situations.

Example

To gain an insight into just how it feels to be "elderly", a nurse disguised herself as an arthritic lady of about 80 years. She proceeded to go shopping and to travel on a bus to find out how she would be treated by society. Her experiences were unpleasant to say the least. The "old lady" was mocked, abused, assaulted and given little or no help in shops and queues and on public transport.

Shortly after her appearances as an old lady the nurse returned, dressed as herself. On each occasion she attempted the same interactions with the same people. Reactions were very different. People smiled, were helpful and happy to make conversation.

During the time she was dressed as an old lady, the nurse felt alone, frightened and sometimes threatened. She felt very angry that many people appeared not to notice the pain, anxiety and helplessness of others.

There were a few people who were nice, and it was noticed that just one person being nice made other people more aware – which defused the atmosphere of irritation and annoyance. (Green 1991)

Health professionals who work with the elderly may often seem more ageist than the general population because they assume that the problems of their clients are typical for all old people. The fact that many of these problems are witnessed over and over again probably does not help. Very often clients' physical problems are dealt with at the expense of their emotional difficulties.

Carers may often make assumptions. This is shown when people talk loudly to anyone over 70, often shouting. The assumption in this case is that everyone over 70 is deaf, and if they are deaf they must be stupid.

There is a tendency to **discriminate** against the elderly, which is in itself an aspect of ageism. Being patronizing, demeaning or displaying derogatory attitudes can often be found within "official" aspects of life. Local authorities, social security pensions offices and the media are often seen to be guilty of portraying these attitudes. Nursing homes and homes for the elderly may also display other examples of discrimination. The elderly in these situations are neatly labelled and

Think about
Reflect on the past few weeks. When you met an elderly person how did you speak? Normally? Loudly? Did you bother to speak at all?

compartmentalized as if they were being put to one side out of the way. Today society abhors the idea of "institutionalization", but there is real danger of institutionalizing the elderly. Sometimes these attitudes go a stage further, edging towards abuse.

Abuse of the elderly

One definition of abuse put forward is: "any act or behaviour by a family member or person providing care (informally or formally) which results in physical or mental harm or neglect of an elderly person" (Podnieks 1985).

Physical abuse includes deliberate inflicting of pain or injury as well as preventing access to health care. **Neglect** includes inattention, abandonment and confinement, and **psychosocial harm** refers to not showing affection, social isolation, and preventing the elderly from making their own decisions. **Exploitation** is also a form of abuse – it may involve using the elderly person's financial resources for the carer's own ends.

It may seem hard to believe that abuse in any form is inflicted upon the frail and infirm, but from studies carried out it appears to be more common than we might expect. In fact, as many as 400 000 old people are suffering.

The reasons for abuse to this extent are not straightforward, but one possible explanation for abuse may be accumulated stress felt by a carer. Family life today has its own fair share of stressors; add to these the responsibility of caring for an elderly person who may be very frail and confused, and the potential for abuse surfaces. Other possible explanations include, a history of family violence, substance abuse by the carer, the change of role or relationship, and the socially disruptive behaviour of the dependants.

Ageism must be included here as a possible reason for abuse. By stereotyping the elderly as being helpless and of little worth, society itself will be slow to intervene. We are members of society and we will grow old too.

Preventing abuse

The most important step is to be alert to the possibility of abuse. Many people are unable to believe that one human being would deliberately abuse another, and because of that they fail to see what is happening. So, **be alert**.

If you believe that someone is being abused, then it is your duty to report this to your senior manager or supervisor. Should you choose to ignore and not to report what you have seen or heard, then you can be considered as an accessory to the abuse.

Another important step is ensuring that everyone involved with the care of an elderly person communicates with each other, and that the formal and informal carers are helped and supported. In some areas a "carers' support group" has proved very worth while. Such a group gives the carers the opportunity to share their problems and difficulties and provides them with a network of people who can help in times of stress.

Practice point
What support systems are in place for formal and informal carers in your local community or work area?

Quality of care

Some people feel that elderly people should not be treated with intensive and expensive medical care, and that this should be given only to the young, where a successful outcome is more likely. There is perhaps an age-related bias by health professionals, but age should be no more of a factor in deciding on active treatment than are HIV, alcoholism, or smoking-related diseases.

There are elderly people who do not wish to undergo aggressive treatment, but that choice must be theirs. Treatment should be given if the person desires it. Above all, there is the right to die with dignity.

Quality of care is perhaps more than anything about **respect**. Respect for older people is no different from respect for anyone else. Respect for individual rights includes:

- involvement in deciding treatments
- participation in the planning of care
- access to aggressive treatment if desired.

The carer can provide quality care that starts from an individual holistic view. Each elderly person has different beliefs, values and needs. The person should be listened to so that his or her views can be taken into account when planning care. Everyone has a need to be listened to. All too often people talk about old people in front of them as though they were not there or were merely an inanimate object. Some might say "He's demented so it doesn't matter". But as the following true example (from *The Lancet*) highlights, appearances are deceptive.

Example

An elderly man was cared for at home for nearly two years by a community nurse called James. In all that time the patient never spoke a word or gave any indication of having any awareness of his surroundings: he was demented. James spent many hours supporting the man's wife as well as giving nursing care to the patient as he became increasingly frail. One evening James and the old lady were at the bedside. Suddenly the old man opened his eyes, took James' hand and quite clearly said: "Thanks, James, for all you have done for me and the missus" – and died.

People also need to be kept informed about what is happening to them. One of the most important things a carer can do is to spend time with the older person. This reinforces the feeling of being valued and encourages the development of trust between the carer and the cared for. The carer can take this opportunity to foster a positive outlook for the individual – achieved through building confidence and being involved. *Everyone wants to feel valued.*

If the carer uses touch at appropriate times this shows a caring attitude, and an interest in the person. Physical contact can be reassuring and further helps in building a trusting relationship.

Think about
What do you think quality of care and caring means? The issue of quality is explored further in Section 3.

Think about

Carers should resist the temptation to "take over" because it is quicker and there is "always far too much else to do". Think about how you might feel if you were always treated as a child. Next time you are assisting elderly clients, try to stop yourself from doing too much for them, and instead work *with* them.

Dignity must be maintained when providing physical care. This means making sure that the client is kept covered as much as possible during any procedures and that the environment is appropriate. This could be simply that the bed space is kept screened, that the bathroom is not draughty. Potentially embarrassing situations (e.g. using the commode or toilet) need to be handled sensitively.

The older person needs to feel useful and involved in his or her own care. By allowing sufficient time, the person may be able to help in washing and dressing even if only putting on one or two items of clothing.

Families and friends also need quality care. They need to be kept informed of what is happening to their loved ones. They should be given the opportunity to visit with flexible visiting times, and as far as possible privacy for the visit. Relatives need time, too, to talk to the professionals and to be listened to. *Supporting the family is an essential part of holistic care.*

Points to remember

- Support workers are an important part of a team approach providing quality of care to the elderly
- The quality of care you provide will be influenced greatly by your own attitudes and beliefs. Your attitudes need to be positive, and your beliefs should be based on fact not fiction.
- Although caring for the elderly can be stressful and exhausting, it is no less fulfilling than caring for any other group of people.

Glossary

Pathological. Indicating a diseased state or condition, e.g. a pathological fracture is a fracture occurring in diseased bone where there has been little or no external trauma.

Dementia. Progressive deterioration of the mental facilities that is irreversible and affects memory, intellect, judgement, personality and emotional control.

Confusion. Disturbed orientation in regard to time, place or person.

Further reading

Redfern. (ed.) (1991), Nursing Elderly People (Churchill Livingstone). This and the following book are useful in that they cover a broad spectrum of physical, psychological and social aspects of caring for the elderly.

Birchenall and Streight. (1993), Care of the Older Adult, 3rd edn (Lippencott).

Green. (1991), "A two-faced society", Nursing Times, 14 August, pages 26–29. This and the following article highlight the negative attitudes by society toward the elderly.

Fox. [1991], "Victims of abuse", Nursing Times, 14 August, pages 30–31. In addition, **Elderly Care Journal** (published by Nursing Standard) every two months covers a range of issues which relate to elderly people. The journal also regularly features articles written by elderly people about aspects of life and care which are of importance to them.

REFERENCES

Green, S. (1991). A two-faced society, *Nursing Times*, 14 August, pp. 26–29.

Podnieks, E. (1985). Elder abuse: it's time we did something about it. *Canadian Nurse*, 81–2, 36–39.

8 | *Learning disabilities*

Paul Evans

The earlier chapters in this section have looked at individuality, its development, and the attitudes, values and beliefs which can have a major impact on a person. Health and how it is perceived have also been discussed.

This chapter continues the theme of valuing individuals and promoting health by examining the care we give to clients with a learning disability. The issues discussed apply not only to those who care for people with a learning disability but also to a wide range of care situations.

The key issues of this chapter are:
- Your own disability.
- What a learning disability consists of
- The philosophy of care
- Living in the community
- Valuing people
- The support worker as an enabler

Our mutual handicap

This chapter links with the O Unit, Y2 and U4a.

‘*Your handicap is great when you come into contact with us, and that increases our handicap. When one of us meets one of you, especially if it is for the first time, we are quite likely to lack many of the skills for successful communication. We may not be able to think of anything appropriate to say, or to put it into the right words, or to control our facial expression. But you also will show a great lack of skill. You will be embarrassed, you won't be able to think of anything to say, you will speak in an inappropriate tone of voice, you will have a wide grin on your face and ask questions without being interested in the answer. The handicap is thus a mutual one. Both of us have difficulty in communicating with and forming relationships with the other.*’

(Williams and Shoultz 1982)

Names and labels

Before we consider anything about people who have been classed as having a **learning disability** it is important that we look at *names*. In the first place, names help us to identify who we are, and secondly they enable others to respond to us.

Consider the names that people use to address you. You will probably have your first (given) name, your surname, your title (Mr, Mrs, Miss or Ms) or names/titles that relate to your job, or even "nicknames". The name or title used will change depending on who you are with. Someone who knows you well may use your first name, someone else your surname with the appropriate title. Generally, we tend not to notice the effects that these various names have on us or the people we encounter. They only become apparent when they become a form of label and stick to the person throughout *all* aspects of their life. Labels have the effect of identifying things in a general way, rather like the labels used on jars on the supermarket shelf.

Labels often make things look similar, even identical. When we use labels to refer to people, this infers that they are all the same. The term "learning disabilities" is a label. It tells you that a person has some difficulty in learning. Although the label is the same for everyone in this group of people, individually they will be as different as you and your next door neighbour. Labels used in this way can sometimes make us miss the vital and essential ingredient, *the person*.

Labels tend to reflect values and attitudes of our society at large. The following list illustrates that labels which have been used to describe people with a learning disability have changed radically over the last century. Some of these terms are now used as *insults*, yet at one time they were included in Acts of Parliament and sanctioned by professionals:

Mild mental handicap	Retarded
Educationally subnormal	Ineducable
High-grade mental defective	Imbecile
Mildly retarded	Profound mental handicap
Feeble-minded	Low-grade mental defective
Moron	Profoundly retarded
Moderate-severe mental handicap	Untrainable
Severely educationally subnormal	Idiot
Medium-grade mental defective	

Despite the problems it is difficult to get away from labels. You may have a label which reflects your job, your marital status, whether you have children or grandchildren, and even your age. The important factor is that most of these labels are *positive*, and they *change* with circumstances during your lifetime. Having a label such as "learning disability" is often *for life*, and for many people this dictates how their life will work out. The effect, as we will see later, is very important.

Think about
When you go to a supermarket, think of how you identify things. Is it the colour of the labels, the sizes of the letters or the words themselves? What happens when the company changes a label? This can make it difficult to find the item unless it has been displayed in a special way.

Think about
How you would feel if someone were to call you subnormal or defective?

What exactly is a learning disability?

The disability is usually something that starts at or around birth, or perhaps in early childhood, and it affects how a person develops intellectually. There *may* be an accompanying physical disability, or a particular set of circumstances or characteristics that the medical profession has identified and given a label to – Down's syndrome for example.

For the majority of people with a learning disability there is no readily identifiable physical reason why they find it difficult to learn at the same speed as others. So, we can identify two major categories:

- physical causation
- social/environmental causation.

Physical causation

Many people belive that a learning disability is due to a physical problem. In reality, physical causation accounts for only one-third of those identified as having a learning disability.

Many physical causes have been given names and are identified as "syndromes" or "conditions" by the medical profession. *It must be remembered, though, that people who have the same syndrome are as different from each other as are people who have the same hair colour or name.* Remember the ideas we looked at on labelling!

Down's syndrome is probably the most widely known syndrome and is the result of a chromosome disorder. Chromosomes are found in every cell in the body. They contain the genes which make us who we are and contribute to the differences between individuals. All human cells should contain 23 pairs of chromosomes, but in Down's syndrome the cells contain 47 rather than 46 chromosomes. This condition is named after John Langdon Down who first described it, and occurs in about 1 in 700 births, although the older a mother is the greater chance of the child being born with this syndrome. Should the mother herself have Down's syndrome, then the chance of the baby being affected rises dramatically to 50%

Antenatal screening is an important aspect of the care we provide for pregnant women, and any woman who is considered to be at risk may be offered a test such as a blood sample or amniocentesis, to find out whether or not the fetus has a chromosome abnormality. Amniocentesis involves obtaining a sample of the amniotic fluid surrounding the fetus and examining the skin cells shed by the fetus. This procedure carries the risk of miscarriage, and should the result be positive there may be a dilemma for the woman and her partner. Termination may be the chosen option but each case must be considered independently.

The abilities of people with Down's syndrome vary enormously, some people being very able and others less so. It is important to highlight that you need to find out what each individual can do and what support will be needed for the thing(s) they find difficulty with. This will be discussed in more detail in the section which looks at the role of the enabler.

Social and environmental causation

In the majority of people for whom a social or environmental factor is the cause, the learning disability is usually quite mild. There is evidence to show that social class is a contributory factor, although not a cause in itself.

In areas where facilities are poor, a combination of factors may lead to susceptible children developing more slowly than others. In some cases this becomes significant enough for the child to be identified as having a learning disability. There are areas in the UK where social and environmental conditions are particularly poor for a variety of reasons, and research has shown that this can markedly affect childrens' performance at school, social interaction and their future adult development.

Where changes have been made to the social conditions people live in, and where improvements have been made in the general health of the population, the knock-on effect has been a raising of the social functioning of those individuals who have been labelled as having a learning disability. This is one of the main reasons why hospitals/institutions have been seen to be inappropriate, and ordinary housing and experiences have begun to replace them. These are factors which both local and national governments are aware of and in some instances have taken steps to rectify, but they are factors that should concern us all.

> ### Point to remember
> What we do know, however, is that each person is an individual in their own right, with the same needs as you or I.

Community care

During the past 20 years, great efforts have been made to develop what has become known as **community care**. One of the first things to consider, when looking at community provision for people with learning disabilities, is that the majority have always lived in the community.

By "community" we tend to mean somewhere you feel you belong, where you meet people you know, where you use facilities that others use and value. Only a small percentage of people (about 10%) have lived in institutions or hospitals and been excluded from their local community. This figure is interesting when you consider the amount of concern that is often focused on hospital closures.

It is estimated that there are approximately one million people in the UK who have a learning disability, so the numbers of these people who have been in hospital could be as few as 100 000. This is the group that society has highlighted, while appearing to ignore the fact that the remaining 900 000 have always been around and living in the community.

Perhaps it is society's fear of these institutions and their reputation that has led to the particular focus being placed on this group of people. In other words, it is fear based upon attitudes and prejudice towards something that many people know little about.

Think about
Using the following list as a guide, consider how each of these factors might influence the ability to learn:
- housing
- transport
- nutrition
- leisure
- hygiene

You may be able to add to this list.

Think about
Why do you think people have prejudices? Is it due to their own intolerance, preconceptions, biases, fear or ignorance?

An ordinary home

It was in Scandinavia that work first began on the integration into mainstream society of people with learning disabilities. In Sweden in the 1960s and 70s, the Board of Health and Welfare developed a number of small residential facilities. The idea was that the small group home approach was the best way to integrate people into local communities. The Board of Health and Welfare were careful in selecting the houses used and chose them in areas within the local community. The houses were home to a relatively small number of people, and this may have helped to foster **positive attitudes** towards those with a learning disability.

At about the same time in Denmark, a National Service for the Mentally Retarded was formed. The philosophy of the service was also one of integration, and aimed to provide a life which was as close to normal as possible. This was the beginning of what we now know as "**normalization**", but it was to take another 10–20 years of development before it became common practice in the UK.

Normalization – a way of relating

It was a man called Wolf Wolfensberger who helped develop the ideas that started off in Scandinavia in the 1960s. Major developments in Nebraska and in other areas in the USA led to some basic but nonetheless powerful principles emerging that have since changed services in the UK in a tremendous way. To understand this fully we need to look at some of the ideas that Wolfensberger (1972) and others developed.

Think about

Think about a group of people who you believe are seen as "less valued" by our society.

▷ What are your ideas about this group?

▷ Include names used with this group, treatment by others, images, and services available.

▷ Compare your thoughts and ideas with those of colleagues.

Can you draw any conclusions as regards how society treats people who are "less valued"?

Point to remember

According to Wolfensberger, normalization is: "The utilization of culturally valued means in order to establish or maintain personal behaviours, experiences and characteristics that are culturally normative or valued."

Normalization applies to people who are seen by a society as being less valued than others. This could apply equally well to the elderly, to those with a mental health problem, to the unemployed, or even to those who have been in prison. The process of being "less valued" occurs when a person is seen as being different, and when the difference is significant enough, society reacts in a negative way.

This negative process begins by our making a value judgement on another individual, but eventually this becomes so strong that the other person begins actually to respond in a way that serves to confirm what we erroneously believed. This is generally known as a "*vicious circle*" (see Figure 8.1).

From Wolfensberger's definition we can begin to see that one of his aims was to use normalization to change the experiences encountered by people who are "less valued".

A vicious circle can be very hard to break, unless those involved with the person can in some way change *their* behaviour or ideas about how they view individuals who have a learning disability. This might lead to a reversal of the

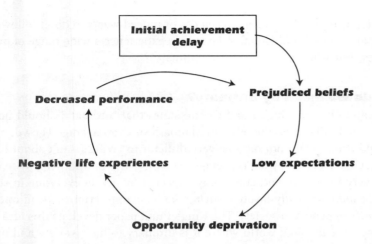

Figure 8.1   A vicious circle (after O'Brien and Tyne 1981)

Think about
Think of someone you know who has a learning disability. Consider a detailed "vicious circle" of their life. How has this been affected by others beliefs and perceptions? From this exercise you may see that, once people begin to respond to someone in a negative way, *everything* the person does seems to justify people's feelings and beliefs.

circumstances that the person who has been "less valued" experiences. Now a "virtuous circle" can be set up (Figure 8.2).

This "virtuous circle" requires you to approach every interaction in a positive way. Look at the person, see what they *can* do and are *good* at, instead of seeing only what they have difficulties with.

You may find it quite difficult to think of all the things *you* can do well, and this may actually say more about our society than about you. We sometimes do not promote ourselves too much in case we are accused of being boastful or bragging. In fact, if we feel that we can do something well, we often feel more positive about ourselves in general. If we use this idea with people who have a learning disability, then we should focus on their strengths and their needs and not their problems.

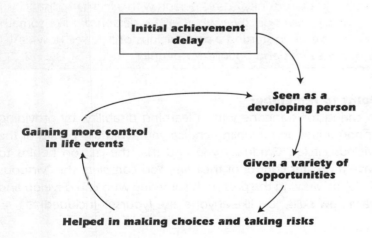

Figure 8.2   A virtuous circle (after O'Brien and Tyne 1981)

Think about
First think about some of the things you can do well (for example drive or swim). Next think about all the things you cannot do. Consider the things you cannot do and imagine that this is the only information people have about you. How do you think others will view you?

By focusing on what a person *can* do, or indeed *wants* to do, it follows that it is necessary for each individual to be able to experience a wide range of **ordinary activities**. But what do we mean by "ordinary"?

What do we mean by ordinary?

A publication by the King's Fund Centre states that "ordinary" should not mean dull or exactly like everyone else, or standard or even average (Lowdon 1980). Such a position would not only be very difficult to create (think about how you would get agreement on what is average); it would also be another way to devalue what is very important and commonly expected by nearly everyone in society.

To be ordinary really involves having the same **opportunities** *and* **options** *as the majority of* people in society. The King's Fund paper develops this idea further by stating: "We live in a world where it is ordinary to have variety and opportunity and choice."

In order to do this, people directly involved with those with learning disabilities need to be able to provide suitable opportunities – not in a haphazard way but in a way which supports the person and enables meaningful choice. Instead of you deciding what someone else wants, you need to present them with a range of options. For this to be successful you obviously need to know the person with whom you are involved extremely well.

Practice point

▶ Choose someone you know and write down a list of their likes and dislikes as far as you know them. This could include their favourite food and drink, places, people or hobbies.

▶ Ask someone else who knows the person well to do the same.

▶ Then ask the person you have chosen to do the same.

▶ What are the similarities and differences in your lists?

The danger in you drawing up a list like this is that you are assuming or guessing what the person may like or dislike. This could result in you withholding an opportunity from a person with a learning disability. In this way you would never discover whether the person did like something, and you could end up starting a new "vicious circle". See how easy it is to reduce opportunities and options for people!

Point to remember

In caring for someone with a learning disability, by providing opportunities and enabling choice you avoid the pitfalls of the "vicious circle". Gradually you find that the person begins to have a greater control of their life. You complete the "virtuous circle" by viewing the person as someone who can develop and learn new skills, just like anyone else (yourself included).

Earlier you were invited to think about the things you have learned to do well. You may have included learning to drive, playing a musical instrument, knitting, cooking or using a computer. Consider now how you learned to do these things? What help did you get? How was it taught? Did you learn it all at once? You may remember that the things you learned to do were broken down into small steps that you could do before you went on to the next stage of learning. You can use this same technique when helping clients with a learning disability, or in any situation where skills need to be relearnt, as in rehabilitation. This is another way to support someone in an opportunity or skill that you have helped them to encounter.

Normalization, then, is a set of principles which guide people and services in a direction that enables those who have been devalued to experience ordinary everyday things so that they can be revalued in mainstream society.

The role of the enabler

If you accept the ideas contained in the principle of normalization, the role of the carer becomes fairly clear. In fact the word "carer" perhaps should not be used in this setting. Caring tends to be seen as something that one person does *to* another. (Remember the "nurturing parent ego state" in Chapter 4.) Indeed, people often talk about being in a *caring relationship*. The role that you take on in your relationship with someone with a learning disability could be better described as an **enabler**. This is because the relationship you have with a person who has a learning disability should be that of an equal, no matter how severe the disability.

The role that you should adopt is that of helping, or enabling, so that the person can achieve things that he or she would have difficulties with without your support. The reason for choosing the word "enabler" (remember what we said about labels) is that it describes exactly what you should be doing.

When you take on the role of carer you may feel pressured into doing everything for the other person. The result is that the person can become dependent on you to do things. In fact he or she can become more disabled as a result. Remember the "vicious circle".

> **Point to remember**
> You should in most cases do the minimum necessary for the person with a learning disability, to enable that person to do the maximum.

This does not mean that you are being lazy – quite the reverse, because to do this effectively is a skill that takes time to develop. The major issue is the relationship you have with the person with the learning disability. This relationship is the most important part of your role as an enabler. Your role should focus on the whole person, and not just a part of him or her. Consider all aspects of life – who they meet with, work with, and their friends outside the home environment.

"Accomplishments"

Normalization can be used as a guide to developing your relationship with your client, but also consider the work by O'Brien and Lyle (1987) which will help you to focus on particularly important areas.

O'Brien and Lyle's **accomplishments**, as they are known, spell out in some detail the aspects of anyone's life which affect their standing in society as a whole. These aspects include

- Dignity
- Respect
- Community presence
- Choice and competence
- Community participation

With regard to **dignity** and **respect**, the role the enabler has to adopt is that of a supporter of the individual. The support should enable the person to fulfil a valued role in the local community. This is actually much easier than it may sound, and can be achieved by the way the enabler relates to individuals with a learning disability. By relating to adults as adults and not as children or second-class citizens, the enabler will provide the individual with the opportunities to respond appropriately. Support is needed to bridge the gap between what the person cannot do at present and what is required of him or her in the future. This shows respect for the needs of the individual and at the same time retains the person's dignity, which would be lost if they were seen to fail.

Community presence means simply mixing with other people within the local community who do not have a learning disability – in a word, **integration** in all aspects of life, including the home setting, daytime activities and leisure pursuits. Segregated groups are not appropriate. Respect and dignity are maintained as people begin to realize just how "able" those with learning difficulties are.

In order to make **choices** and become **competent** in everyday skills, the person with a learning disability has to be presented with the opportunities and experiences in which to make a choice and become competent. (Remember the vicious and virtuous circles.) Providing an individual with the opportunity to make a decision is something which will continue to influence him or her throughout life. The decisions do not have to be major ones at first, but may simply start with a decision on whether to have tea or coffee. With further support and encouragement, the major decisions – such as where to live, who to live with and what job to undertake – will be made more easily. Obviously, each individual needs a different level of support. As the person gradually gains confidence and skills, this is turn will encourage others to view him or her in a more positive light.

As decision-making skills develop, so too will the respect and dignity afforded by others, and a change may occur in the degree of integration or community presence too. *The virtuous circle will emerge.*

Finally, under **community participation** the enabler must take into account the rights of the individual not only to live, work and socialize in the local community, but also to be free to build relationships with others – to have

Think about
What reasons are given when people or groups are segregated?

friends of his or her choosing and to have contact with relatives in an unimpeded and relaxed manner. Friendships need not be limited to platonic ones. People with a learning disability have the right to meaningful relationships, which may include sexual relationships, the opportunity to marry and have children of their own.

Think about

Think about your own attitude to the idea of people with a learning disability integrating fully into the community and having intimate relationships. Be honest with yourself, but bear in mind the vicious circle and identify how easily you can restrict an individual's rights and opportunities.

You might find it helpful to talk through this idea with a friend or colleague.

As an enabler you will need to put these ideas into practice, but your knowledge of the individual can be used alongside your knowledge and understanding of the facilities and services available in your area.

Points to remember

- We are all disabled in some way. None of us is perfect. We are all aware that there is something we have difficulty with or feel we cannot do.
- With help we could overcome our disability, and in the same way so can people with a learning disability.
- The process of *integration* has a number of knock-on effects. It can highlight to others that people with a learning disability *can achieve* and *can develop* just like you and I.

Practice activity

With a friend, a pair of rubber gloves and a blindfold, try to do some of the tasks you do every day. Put the rubber gloves and blindfold on yourself. Your friend can only talk you through the tasks. Examples of things to do include: threading a bobbin, tying your shoelaces, pouring a drink. After the exercise discuss how you would make the task easier, so you could do it without being frustrated. Imagine how a person with a learning disability might feel if they encountered problems like this every day. Many people do!

Further reading

Clark. (1982), Mentally Handicapped People Living and Learning (Baillière Tindall).

Potts and Fido. (1991), A Fit Person to be Removed (Northcote). A graphic insight into what life was like in an institution, and an understanding of why there has been a move by the caring profession to close hospitals for people with a learning disability.

Ryan and Thomas. (1987), The Politics of Mental Handicap (Free Association

Books). Looks at the politics and real-life issues surrounding the lives of people with a learning disability.

Shanley and Starrs. (1993), Learning Disabilities – A Handbook of Care, 2nd edn (Churchill Livingstone). A useful all-round book covering a wealth of issues, including causation and normalization. Recommended as a foundation textbook for Project 2000 courses.

Towell and Beardshaw. (1991), Enabling Community Integration (Kings Fund Centre). Takes some of the points mentioned here a step further and looks at practical realities.

REFERENCES

Lowdon K.F.C. (1980). *An Ordinary Life: Comprehensive Local Services for Mentally Handicapped People*, Kings Fund Centre.

O'Brien J. and Lyle C. (1987). *Framework for Accomplishment*, Responsive System Association (Decator, Georgia).

O'Brien J. and Tyne A. (1981). *The Principles of Normalization – A Foundation for Effective Services*, Campaign for Mentally Handicapped People (London).

Williams P. and Shoultz B. (1982). *We Can Speak For Ourselves*, Souvenir Press.

Wolfensberger W. (1972). *The Principles of Normalization in Human Service*, National Institute on Mental Retardation (Downsview, Toronto).

SECTION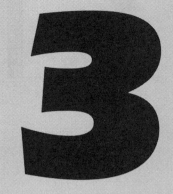

Quality in care

Introduction

Quality is about high standards, about legal and moral values, about responsibility, and about safety. Quality in care is more than "doing no harm" to the client – it is about using your practical caring skills to the optimum standard through knowledge and understanding.

There have been many discussions around accountability, and professional carers such as doctors, nurses and physiotherapists all have governing bodies to which they are accountable. These bodies have the power to discipline and suspend practitioners who fail to practise within the guidelines laid down in their codes of conduct.

Although support workers do not have such a code of conduct, they are still accountable under the laws of the land in which they work, both for the standard and for the quality of care they give. This section of the book considers a number of areas which are of huge importance to all support workers practising in any care situation.

Competence is not just the ability to carry out a practical skill. It is also about being able to recognize the complexities of holistic care within an organizational framework. Additionally it is equally important to understand oneself, one's abilities and limitations of knowledge and role. You should know the boundaries in which you must work.

The five chapters are linked by standards of responsibility which apply to the quality of care and safety of clients, their friends and relatives, and everyone who is a part of the organization.

9 Putting quality into perspective

Angela Turner

This chapter addresses the subject of quality assurance (QA). This is an issue that has particular relevance for everyone involved in caring for others. The primary objective is for you to develop a basic grasp of quality assurance and its application to health care delivery.

Subjects specifically associated with quality include the Patient's Charter, standards, complaints and audit. You may already be familiar with some of these, but help in developing the skills and the practicalities of implementation within the workplace is a gap frequently expressed by health care workers.

The key issues of this chapter are:
- Defining quality
- Client interest and support groups
- Health care reforms
- The Patients' Charter
- Complaints
- Patient satisfaction monitoring
- Standards
- Audit
- Quality and your role

Introducing quality

Quality in the health care setting is regarded as a fairly new concept. It is difficult to say when the subject of quality was seen to be particularly important. Some argue that quality has always been at the forefront of care, others say that quality only became topical with the introduction of general management in the mid-1980s. Despite the disagreement about its beginnings, what is apparent is that quality is here to stay and concerns us all.

This chapter links with Core Unit O, U4 and Y2.

Defining quality

Explaining the meaning of quality often proves to be a troublesome task, because no single definition exists. One well-known and often deliberated definition is expressed as "I know quality when I see it, but I can't explain it." Another plausible explanation is that quality is "**cost-related**". Quality and cost are very often linked. When buying a car, an assumption is made that the more you pay the better the car; a less expensive version will still get you from A to B but not necessarily in the style or comfort that a more expensive model would allow.

However, we need to be careful about making a simple link between cost and quality. Quality is cost-related – but if we return to the analogy of the car, we need also to consider performance, reliability, safety and after-sales service, which are all indicative of quality. Quality therefore covers a wide range of issues, not just the initial cost.

Health care costs many millions of pounds to provide. Many questions are being asked about how the National Health Service can give a quality service, and value for money. This chapter explores some of the points where we can make the quality of health care clearer and how we might ensure value for money.

Media interest

We often read in our daily newspaper (or hear on the television or radio) how marvellous the National Health Service (NHS) is. We are told of dedicated people working long hours with little reward. At least this used to be the case. The public perception of health care is changing, with the focus shifting from staff and conditions to the actual care given.

An indication of this change in focus is demonstrated by the development of **league tables** which attempt to show how well (or otherwise) health care establishments are doing. In particular these tables show figures associated with the **Patients' Charter** (1991). An example is consultants' waiting lists – that is, how long a person has to wait from referral by their GP to their appointment in a clinic with the consultant.

Public interest in league tables is growing, and you may already be aware of the league tables associated with the general education system. Clients of the NHS are led to believe that league tables are indicative of the quality of care available, but they form only part of a very large quality equation.

Some argue that it is a good thing that hospitals have to publish this sort of information because it provides the public with an opportunity to compare performances. Potentially, this is a cause for concern. A balance needs to be made between those activities that are easy to count, such as day cases and outpatient department waiting times, and those that are not easy to count. The difficulty in creating a balance is discussed further in this chapter.

Client interest and support groups

Client interest can be expressed through support groups, whose influence can and does affect how health care is delivered. This applies to *primary* and *secondary* care.

Support groups have had an enormous effect on the delivery and quality of client care. The last 15 years have seen a steady increase in differing specialist groups, all with a vested interest in securing the best possible care for their

Think about
What does quality mean to you and your family? How would you define quality?

Think about
Are you familiar with
the Community Health
Council or the
Candelighters Group?
The primary objective
of these groups is to
represent clients' views.
Are you aware of any
other patient or client
groups and do you
know their functions?

particular group. Examples are Age Concern, Mencap, the Cancer Support Group and the National Childbirth Trust.

Expanding on quality

We could argue that quality is about *everything* we do, and if we subscribe to this ideal then quality is more than "hands on" client care at the bedside. Quality concerns all of us, every day. Quality of information (for example, clarity, legibility, and accuracy); how we communicate, verbally and non-verbally, with one another; how we act; how we portray ourselves; these are all indicative of the quality of the service we give.

To illustrate further the simplicity of quality, consider the following true example.

Example

A client was being wheeled on a trolley by a porter to the operating theatre. The client asked what quality meant to the porter. After a short pause he replied: "Missing the bumps on the corridor."

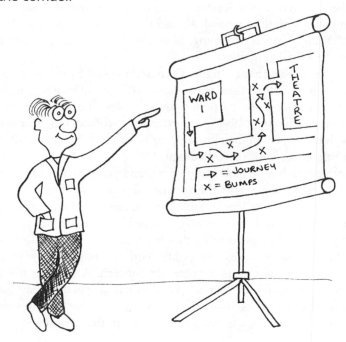

This small gesture was a huge contribution to client comfort, and care is overwhelmingly what quality is about. Care for others in a way that you would wish for yourself and for members of your family.

Already many aspects of quality are beginning to emerge and what is actually involved. It is influenced by:

- value for money
- individuals and teams
- communication
- media interest and public perceptions

The issue of quality can be seen to be far-reaching, and its application should wherever possible be kept as simple as possible.

Health care reforms

There have been numerous reforms of the way the National Health Service is provided since its inception in 1948. The most recent reforms have given health care providers, such as hospitals, much more control over how they deliver care to the community in which they are based. **Trusts**, like any other business, have to balance the books and compete with others for contracts of care. Every NHS Trust will want to give its customers the best. Clients, and those purchasing care on clients' behalf, will need assurance that the quality of care will be of a high standard.

Making quality clear and explicit, and ensuring that patients and clients receive the best possible care within the resources available, has been a major component of government reforms. The Patients' Charter added impetus to making quality explicit.

The Patients' Charter

The Charter sets out national and local **standards** for hospitals to meet. The standards in the Charter have certainly had an impact. Hospitals are bound to ensure that the standards are implemented and that they are monitored on a quarterly basis.

Possibly the best known example of quality is "waiting times" in the out-patient department. The Charter standard states that you will be given a specific appointment time and be seen within 30 minutes of that time.

Clients do have to wait, and some delays are inevitable for many reasons. However, if they are kept waiting then a simple and courteous explanation must be given. Clients can be given a variety of options so they can select an appropriate course of action suitable for them. Some will continue to wait, others may choose to return later, others may wish to rearrange their appointment.

You can imagine a department where a lot of clients are kept waiting without explanation. The nurses and doctors are busy and the tension between the waiting clients and the staff increases. Communication breaks down and clients complain.

However, we need to exercise caution when linking the quality of care with the efficiency of the organization. Quality is not only about "waiting", although the two are often linked together. Quality is also about the *consultation itself* –

Think about
When you experience "waiting" for a bus or a train, how do you feel?

Think about
How would you feel if you were kept waiting or felt "processed" without consideration to your feelings, fears and questions? Would you make a complaint if you were unhappy with the service?

whether the client has understood what was being said and agreed with the course of treatment and/or care, and whether the client considered that he or she was treated like a human being rather than being "processed" like a can of peas. So, although league tables form part of the quality picture, the most important aspect of quality is the **interaction** that takes place between health care staff and the client. It is the exchange of information and how that information is communicated that makes for a successful consultation. Some clients need to be given more time than others to assimilate what is being said, to enable them to make an informed choice about their care and treatment.

Point to remember
It is all very well to say that an efficient outpatient department will have the majority of clients seen within a given time. If the consultations are rushed the clients may leave the hospital or clinic confused and upset. How can that be considered a quality service?

Complaints
Some people are quite capable of articulating their feelings, others find it very difficult. A few may think "Why bother?". So one person who does complain is probably speaking for 10 or more people who for some reason do not. So why do clients not complain as often as they could – what makes it difficult for them to complain?

The situation is not hard to understand. We do know that as a race the British in particular tend not to complain, but evidence suggests that this too is changing.

All hospitals and community services (this applies to both the public and the private sectors) are required to have a **complaints procedure** in place. Hospital and community trusts must publish their complaints to their purchasing authorities on a quarterly basis.

The Patients' Charter states that any client has the right "to have any complaint about NHS services – whoever provides them – investigated and to receive a full and prompt reply from the Chief Executive or General Manager".

Quite apart from the complaints procedure, are complaints (or the shortage of them) indicative of the quality of the service being given? We have to be aware that the majority of clients will not complain even when they feel aggrieved.

The whole subject of complaints is very emotive. Often the staff involved will feel negative and undervalued if a complaint is made about them or about the services they have provided. Not all complaints are justified and staff need to be reassured accordingly. However, there are circumstances where complaints *are* justified, and the appropriate action needs to be taken. One Regional Manager has suggested that we should treat complaints as "nuggets of gold" and consider them all a **learning experience** for individuals and the organization.

Think about
▶ As a client, would you know *how* to complain and *to whom*?
▶ As a member of the care staff, what would be your actions if a client complained to you?

Patient satisfaction monitoring
People have in the past tended to tolerate a poor service of any kind, not just on health-related matters. We have all no doubt accepted such a situation rather than

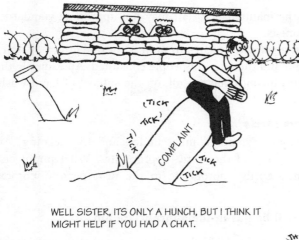

WELL SISTER, ITS ONLY A HUNCH, BUT I THINK IT
MIGHT HELP IF YOU HAD A CHAT.

cause a fuss. Only by asking questions of those to whom a service is being supplied do we begin to find out how acceptable the service is.

It is extremely important for all organizations to listen to their customers. Health care workers can learn a lot by observing how shops, hotels and restaurants treat their consumers, and how the emphasis is changing from what an organization wants to supply, to a customer-led service. This interesting change is now occurring in the National Health Service. Clients' views on the service are actively being sought, and a lot of literature has been published. Should you wish to explore this further, ask for help from your supervisor as there are a number of important issues such as **confidentiality** and **ethics** that can make patient satisfaction monitoring complicated.

Making quality explicit through standards

One way in which we can contribute to making quality explicit is through the writing and developing of **standards**. Standards can be grouped into subject areas. Examples are:

- *professional standards*, which are laid down by professional bodies such as the United Kingdom Central Council (UKCC) for Nursing, Midwifery and Health Visiting.
- *clinical standards* for medical and nursing practice
- *environmental standards*, dealing for example with cleanliness of operating theatres, heating, lighting, ventilation
- *educational standards* as laid down by the professional bodies to ensure that all professional health care workers maintain their competence.

Put simply, a standard is "an agreed level of performance" that is written by and for those to whom it applies. It is important that groups of staff developing the standards do so for their practice, and not for the practice of others! Despite best intentions, the maintenance staff may not appreciate standards written for them by receptionists.

Obviously, if a standard relates to more than one group of staff then advice needs to be sought and the relevant people consulted. An example that applies to us all is a standard for *infection control*, on the subject of hand-washing.

Clarity of standards

Everyone who reads a standard must understand its meaning. An ambiguity frequently arises by use of the word "appropriate". What might be appropriate to you is not necessarily appropriate to the next person. For example, if a standard states:

All sharps will be put in the appropriate bin

the words "appropriate bin" could mean any form of receptacle. ("Sharps" are defined as needles, blades or any object that is sharp and may cause an injury or infection if not disposed of correctly). A new member of staff, for instance, could interpret this as an ordinary waste-paper bin. Staff who removed the waste from clinical areas might end up with a serious injury which could have been avoided. Reworded, the statement reads:

All sharps will be disposed of in a sharps box.

The reader of the standard will now understand that the receptacle is more than just an ordinary waste bin. The standard expresses explicitly how the disposal is to take place.

To make the writing of standards easier, the mnemonic "rumba" is often applied. That is, a standard should be:

> **r**eliable (always achieves same results)
> **u**nderstandable (clear and unambiguous)
> **m**easurable (have a known value on a scale)
> **b**ehavioural (there is an observable response)
> **a**chievable (the defined target can be reached).

Auditing by means of criteria

The most frequent problem people have with standards is how to review and evaluate (**audit**) them.

We have seen that the *standard statement* is the level of performance to be achieved. Further actions are required to uphold the statement. These further actions are referred to as **criteria**. There may be one or two or several criteria – this depends on the subject. These criteria are then turned into questions.

Example

The standard on the topic of infection control might look like this (note that in your own care setting the standard might be different):

Topic: Infection control

Standard statement: All sharps will be disposed of in a sharps box.

Criteria:

1. Sharps boxes will be available in all clinical areas.
2. Sharps boxes will be clearly labelled.
3. Sharps boxes will be colour-coded

For ease of use, the standard statement and the criteria would be on one sheet of paper and the audit questions would be on a separate or second page. The audit looks like this:

1. Are sharps boxes available in all clinical areas?   YES/NO
2. Are all sharps boxes clearly labelled?   YES/NO
3. Are all sharps boxes colour-coded?   YES/NO

A simple calculation – adding the number of "yes" responses together – will show whether you have achieved the standard or not.

Sometimes you may find that a criterion is simply not applicable ("N/A"). It might, for example, be considered unsafe to have a sharps box in a clinical area where clients could inflict deliberate self-harm. Therefore "N/A" may be a legitimate response.

If problems arise and the staff cannot achieve the standard, it might be that the standard is set unrealistically high. Basic minimum standards should be achievable. Therefore an agreement between the practitioners and the supervisors is sought to determine the level of acceptability. Sometimes it is of value to involve clients and their carers in setting standards, but it is important to emphasize that improvement is the overall aim of standards. There is little point in being unrealistic. It is better to start by knowing what can be achieved and then to try to make the necessary improvements.

How many standards?

The ideal number of standards a department should have is difficult to ascertain. Clearly, to have lots of standards implies a lot of time auditing them. It really does depend on the area of the service as to how many should be developed. It is up to the staff to develop as many as they think necessary. A word of caution – do not try to write a huge number of standards in order to gain a competitive advantage over your colleagues, without first demonstrating that your existing standards are working! Experience has shown that ten or so good reliable standards are effective and beneficial to begin with. The more standards, the more auditing. Be realistic, start small and then grow.

Point to remember

Make sure you understand the differences between *policies*, *procedures* and *standards*. If necessary ask your supervisor to help you.

Think about
What subjects could you contribute to? Could you develop standards for support workers in your area?

Standards really can be interesting! They help you to clarify what you are trying to achieve, and they help to explain to others what you are trying to do.

Practice point

You could publish your results in your area of work, and perhaps compare a past audit with a recent one. Have you made progress? If you have only a low score, look upon this positively and try to improve for the next audit.

Look to another area. Have they written a standard on the same topic? Can you learn from them?

Audit and change

The final component of this chapter concerns audit of treatment and care. This is the process of analysing data to establish what treatment or care has been given, and whether it actually did what it was supposed to do.

An audit may take place after an event has occurred, and this is called **retrospective audit** (e.g. after discharge from hospital or care). **Prospective audit** is carried out as care is delivered (e.g. wound care). A further simple example of restrospective audit would be a questionnaire for a client to complete concerning various aspects of their care or treatment regime. The data are then analysed and if any negative areas are highlighted a plan is drawn up to address any deficits.

Auditing is a cyclical process. First we observe clinical practice – what is actually happening. Secondly we move on a stage and ask ourselves whether this is what we want to happen: "Should this practice be occurring?". Thirdly, if the described practice is not being carried out, change is implemented. In reality the first two steps are not too difficult to achieve. The third stage – implementing changes to practices – can be very difficult, especially if staff feel threatened or intimidated by change.

The idea of change can be very difficult for individuals to accept, especially if they cannot perceive the changes to be beneficial to either themselves or client care. Change has to be handled very sensitively and with compassion. It is not something that will happen overnight, but will require a lot of effort by everyone involved.

In 1986 the government published *Working for Patients*, part of which is concentrated on **medical audit**. Medical audit is carried out by doctors. In 1993 a further publication from the Department of Health, *Clinical Audit*, changed the emphasis from a medical to a multiprofessional dimension. **Clinical audit** "involves looking systematically at procedures used for diagnosis, care and treatment, examining how associated resources are used, and investigating the effect of care on the outcome and quality of life for the patient". The change from medical to clinical audit was to ensure that the various professional groups could work collaboratively to improve patient care.

You now need to reflect on your role and your personal contribution to promoting and sustaining quality.

Think about

How often have you heard the comment "I've always done it this way and it works, so why should I change?"

Think about your contribution to delivering a quality service. Can you influence the quality of care?

Points to remember

Think about
Does clinical audit
occur in your area of
work?

■ The singular most important aspect of quality delivery is attitude, and that means the attitude of everyone involved in caring.
■ Quality is not the same as efficiency.
■ Quality can be as simple as a smile or holding someone's hand. Just showing that you are concerned is all that might be required. Your contribution would then have been enormous for that individual.

Glossary

Primary care. The care given to individuals in the community at the first point of contact with the primary health care team. First contact may be with the GP, district nurse or health visitor.

Secondary care. The level in the health care system that consists of emergency treatment and care. Also called "acute care".

Further reading

Oakland. (1993), *Total Quality Management*, 2nd edn (Butterworth–Heinemann). This book is useful for references.

Ovretveit. (1992), *Health Service Quality* (Blackwell Scientific).

DoH. (1994), *The Evolution of Clinical Audit* (Health Publications Unit).

REFERENCES

Department of Health. (1989). *Working for Patients* (HMSO).

Department of Health. (1991). *The Patients' Charter* (HMSO).

Department of Health. (1993). *Clinical Audit* (HMSO).

10 | *Legal aspects of care*

Pamela Bradley

For support workers, the need to consider law in a health care setting may not always be apparent. Law, however, is a discipline which impinges on everyone's life by virtue of its real impact or its perceived threat.

No one is outside the law. As a support worker in any health care setting it is expected that you will comply with the law in the same way as anyone else, both within the workplace and whilst off duty. The law exists to protect the rights of individuals against infringement by another, and provides some order and stability to society.

As a health care worker you have a duty to uphold the rights of individuals and to behave, at all times, in a manner which is in accordance with the privileged position you hold.

The key issues of this chapter are:
- The legal framework
- Health and safety at work
- Confidentiality
- Duties and role of the support worker
- Complaints
- Accidents
- Consent

A privileged position

The general public still appears to believe that all health care workers (particularly those dealing directly with clients) are "special" and holds them in high regard. You may have heard comments such as:

> *"I don't know how you can stand to work in a hospital."*
> *"I think you are all angels."*

This chapter links with the O Unit, U5 and U4.

It is important to be aware of these impressions. Although we all like to let our hair down at times, it is worth remembering that how we conduct ourselves in public may have some bearing on how people see us professionally.

The role of a support worker embraces a degree of **privilege** which in turn carries special **responsibilities**. The support worker must always remember that this privileged position means access to people, their property, their home and personal information. Therefore, respect and regard for each is of paramount importance.

The legal framework

The law of the land comprises criminal law and civil law, and the latter includes employment legislation.

Under **criminal law**, a crime is an offence against the state, either by doing something which the law forbids or by omission of some act which the law requires. Theft is a crime; driving a car without a licence is an omission but still a crime and penalized by a fine or imprisonment.

Civil law is concerned with the rights and duties individuals have towards each other. Legal action may be taken by a private individual against another individual or organization. Much of a health professional's work comes within the framework of civil law. Within this framework there is a part known as the **law of torts** ("omission" in Scotland) which relates to negligence, trespass to the person or assault and battery, and defamation either as libel or slander.

Employment legislation relates to protection of the individual employee and the regulation of industrial relations between employers and employees. Additionally, hospital and community service also has its own "law" laid down by senior officers in conjunction with many other staff, and presented as **policies and procedures**. These are put together to protect both you and your client and to provide a framework for working practices.

Health and safety at work

The legal obligations of employer and employee can best be illustrated by the Health and Safety at Work Act 1974. Of all the laws that apply to health care workers in the UK, this Act is the one which most noticeably affects daily work. Many policies are based on this Act, and many procedures are written to protect the health and safety of employees and clients while outlining standards of care.

By law, employers *must* have a written safety policy, and they must take appropriate action to ensure the health and safety at work of all employees.

Point to remember
By law, every employee must read the safety policy and adhere to it. **This means you!** It is not an option, but a legal requirement of employment. There should be a copy of the safety policy readily accessible to all staff in every unit, department, ward, health centre, community home and so on.

Inhouse "laws" (the policies and procedures) are for all staff, who have personal responsibility to ensure that they work within these written guidelines. Support workers are strongly advised to ensure that they are familiar

Think about
Think about someone you particularly respect or rely upon, like a policeman or a teacher. How would you feel if you saw them dancing on the table of the local pub, or being involved in a public brawl? Would you feel the same respect for them the following day?

with the policies and procedures which apply to their work and organization, and to observe them at all times. This includes wearing a uniform or other protective clothing where provided, responding to emergency signals such as fire alarms, and developing a "safety-conscious" attitude to work. Common policy areas include:

- infection control
- lifting and handling
- drug control
- recruitment and selection
- COSHH (control of substances hazardous to health)

- equal opportunities
- no smoking
- discipline and grievances

Common procedures include:

- admission
- discharge

- handling complaints
- acts following the death of a client

There may also be a range of procedures which relate to particular medical or surgical treatments.

Working in the community

If you are working in the community you may be on your own and colleagues will not be close at hand to assist and advise if anything goes wrong.

If you damage any property whilst working in the community, your employer will be vicariously liable (under the principle of "master and servant") to make good any damage. Should you be at fault because you have failed to take the necessary precautions, then you might be disciplined, by your employer.

Confidentiality

What does "confidential" mean? Most dictionary definitions will include the word "trust".

Confidentiality of information comprises a major part of the National Occupational Standards, which specify the quality of performance required in the workplace. The clients you care for have a right to expect that any information they give about themselves will be used only for the purposes for which it is given. Information should be disclosed or accessible only to people immediately involved in the client's care. Even when a client has died, the obligation to retain confidentiality remains.

Anything you learn about a client in the course of your work is confidential. You are entrusted to maintain that confidentiality. There is no harm in discussing a client's care provided the discussion is held in an appropriate place and with the appropriate people – this generally means in the workplace and only with those who are involved with the client's care.

Confidentiality covers both the written and the spoken word. When answering telephone enquiries it is difficult to be certain of the identity of the caller, so

Think about

Imagine that you are making a call at a house and two large, apparently vicious, dogs are in the garden. Should you risk injury by entering?

If you could not attract the attention of the occupants, then it would be better that you miss the appointment rather than be savaged by dogs. Obviously, on being unable to gain access your supervisor must be informed immediately.

Think about
How would you feel if you learnt that very personal information about you had been discussed in a pub?

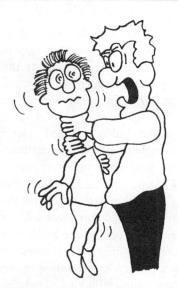

'CONFIDENTIALITY YOU SAID,' - WELL I WENT TO THE PUB QUIZ LAST NIGHT - AND YOU KNOW WHAT THE QUESTIONS WERE ON - ME!

care is needed not to give confidential information. Wherever you work, ensure that you are familiar with the organization's policy on confidentiality and that you seek guidance from your supervisor if in any doubt.

Within health care, the use of computers is rapidly becoming more wide-spread. Rules governing the use and disclosure of information on a database are similar to those for other more conventional records. It should be shared only with people directly involved with the client, and cover only information that is necessary for the purpose for which it is gathered. All information stored in a computer which relates to an individual who can be identified, directly or indirectly, is covered by the Data Protection Act 1984.

There are certain circumstances, however, when confidentiality has to be breached. One occasion may be when a court orders the disclosure of information. Should you refuse to comply with the order, then the court can hold you in contempt – the penalty for which may be a fine or imprisonment.

Another circumstance is in relation to **notifiable diseases** (for example, measles, meningitis) where, despite the client's wishes with regard to confidentiality, notification must be made to the correct authority.

Point to remember

Great care is needed to protect confidentiality. Particular care is needed if you are working within an accident and emergency department. Journalists and police officers may, for example, ask you whether a person's injuries might have been caused by a blow from a hammer or blunt instrument. Should you receive a request of this nature, do not offer an opinion but immediately refer the matter to your supervisor.

Sometimes the police will make a blanket request such as: "Please give me the names and addresses of all males between the ages of 18 and 20 years who have been treated in the last 24 hours for lacerations to the forearm." This type of request is not one to which you are required to respond, and again the matter must be referred to your superior/senior nurse who will no doubt enlist the help of the legal department.

Thinking about the "greater public interest" can cause difficulty. What should you do when you have been given information in confidence and, by maintaining that confidence, you place another person in jeopardy? If, for example, a person confesses to you that he has injured someone and intends to finish the job off on getting out of hopsital, where do you stand with regard to confidentiality? In those circumstances you must ask yourself whether greater harm will be done by breaching the confidence or by maintaining it.

The **public interest** is taken to mean the interests of an individual, group of individuals or society as a whole. It certainly encompasses matters such as serious crime, child abuse and drug trafficking. There is no magic formula for dealing with such events, but by always referring the matter to an appropriate professional you will ensure that the correct procedures are followed.

Access to health records

Within the Patients' Charter, every citizen has a right to have access to their health record, and to know that those working for the NHS will, by law, keep the contents confidential. In general terms, from November 1991 the Access to Medical Records Act allows a client who applies under the terms of the Act to see his or her medical records, subject to specific exceptions.

This applies only to medical records that have been compiled since the Act was introduced, and is not retrospective.

Keeping good records

All health professionals and support workers must be very careful about **documentation**. If what you write is clear, concise, accurate and factual, then you need have no fears. However, it would be wise not to be careless in writing records or reports, and to ensure that anything you do write is capable of substantiation and is signed and dated.

DO'S
- Use black ink.
- Write legibly and indelibly.
- Be clear and unambiguous.
- Be accurate in each entry as to date and time.
- Score out alterations with a single line followed by your signature, date and time of corrected entry.
- Use your full signature.

DON'TS
- Do not use initials.
- Do not use abbreviations or meaningless phrases.
- Do not use pencil or blue ink.
- Do not use any chemical to erase or obscure an entry.

The importance of clear and concise record-keeping cannot be stressed too strongly. Not only is a medical or nursing record the only point of reference for someone to check the condition of a client, medication and related issues; it is also the only point of reference for a member of staff if he or she is ever called to question on what was done at a particular date and time. It is all too easy to assume that you will remember the incident or circumstance. You may well do so for a short period, but some days later the memory will have faded and the recollection will have gone.

Records must always be factual, clear and concise, recording only the exact detail of what has been seen or heard and what action has been taken. When other people are involved, record their full name and status.

It is surprising just how often the date and signature are missing from documentation. Unless something unusual takes place you may have difficulty remembering one client over another, and this will become even more difficult as time passes.

It is useless to make a record which is neither clear nor concise. Read over carefully what you have written, then ask yourself if the colleague who follows you on the next shift will be in any doubt about the meaning of what you have recorded.

Point to remember

Clear, concise and factual records mean that there will be understanding and therefore no misinterpretation.

Example

12 June 94   14.30 hrs
In accordance with the care plan, Mrs Jones has been assisted with an immersion bath. It was noted that her toenails were rough and require cutting. As she is a diabetic, Staff Nurse Allen has been informed and arranged for the chiropodist to visit on 14 June at 10.00 hrs.   *M. Collings*

Giving clear instructions

In health care, as in all other services, it is imperative that instructions, whether they be verbal or written, are given in such a way that there is no risk of misinterpretation.

If you are asked to do something you must be absolutely sure that you understand fully what is being asked of you. If you are in any doubt about the validity of the instruction or your ability to carry it out, then do not hesitate to say so immediately. It would be unwise – and possibly dangerous – to attempt to carry out a task without fully understanding the instruction.

Complaints

The health service receives its fair share of complaints, and all health authorities should have agreed policies and procedures for dealing with them.

If you are involved with a complaint you may be asked to write a "statement of events". Simply write what you know. Do not exaggerate or invent incidents, and if you cannot remember then say so. Do not blame someone else, since there may be a very good reason why they acted in the way they did.

Many people have concerns about writing statements. If you are at all unsure then talk to your immediate manager, senior nurse or union steward. Always ascertain:

- where and to whom the statement is to go
- how the statement is to be used.

Always keep a copy of what you have written.

Example
Mrs Jones' relatives have filed a complaint about the condition of her feet and are concerned that there has been a lack of care and attention:

16 June 94   09.00 hrs

Statement by Maureen Collings, Care Assistant, Rosewood House
On 12 June 1994, my colleague Rani Tingh and I escorted Mrs Jones to the bathroom and proceeded to assist her with an immersion bath, in accordance with the care plan. While washing Mrs Jones I noted that her toenails were long and very rough. I explained to her that I would inform the staff nurse and arrangements would be made for the chiropodist to attend. On completion of the bathing I recorded in the clients notes the state of Mrs Jones's nails and that I had informed the staff nurse.   M. Collings

Point to remember
Clients and their carers who feel that they have a complaint have a right to receive an explanation of the events which have taken place. Should we be in the wrong, then we must be prepared to say so.

Justifiable complaints should always be used in a constructive way to help improve the service we give to clients. More detail is given with regard to complaints in Chapter 9 on Quality.

Accidents
An organization's policy will refer to the procedure to be followed in the event of an accident happening to a client, a visitor or an employee. Many workplaces,

however, have a separate accident procedure. As with the safety policy, following the accident procedure is not an option – *it is a legal requirement.*

Everyone at work has a duty to take care, not only for their own safety but also for the safety of others.

When you have received training in safe lifting techniques, do adhere to that training and do not be tempted to short-cut the system in an attempt to save time or effort. You only have one back and once you have strained it to a degree where it is worthless then your career in caring will be jeopardized.

If you witness a dangerous occurrence, notice a hazard such as a torn piece of carpet, or observe a fault in a piece of equipment, you have a legal responsibility to report it to your employer or departmental manager. If you, a client or a visitor have an accident at work, however trivial it may appear, you must by law report it using the local accident reporting procedure. Take particular care when carrying beverages or other liquids because it is so easy to spill a drop on the floor – a drop which may be no danger to a fit and healthy person but which may result in serious harm by way of a slip or fall to someone who is not particularly steady. Do not use equipment that you are not trained or competent to use, and never use any machinery unless all the necessary guards are in place.

Follow the advice given under "Complaints" if you are asked to make a "statement of events" following an accident in your area of work.

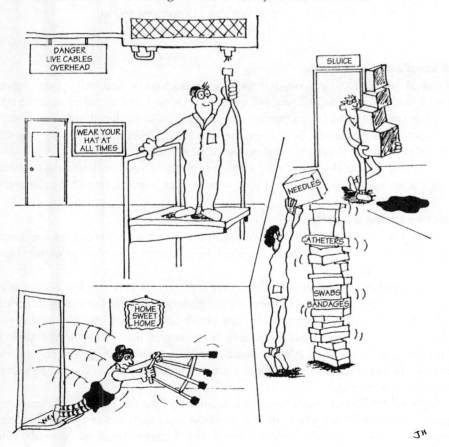

The completed accident form may form part of the legal case (as evidence) if the accident victim – which could be you – should seek to sue the employer for damages. It is vitally important, therefore, that it is fully and accurately completed as soon as possible after an accident occurs.

Duties as a support worker

During your period of training you will have been assessed as competent in various activities. The breadth of these activities will be dependent on the level of training undertaken. The general public with whom you deal are entitled, therefore, to be treated with the degree of competency commensurate with your level of training.

Should you fail to come up to the mark, then you might well be judged to have been negligent under the law and your actions could lead to a claim for damages. Your employer might "pay the bill", but the employer would investigate the events and disciplinary action could follow.

Point to remember
Managers should expect you to work only within your competency levels, but you yourself have a duty **not** to undertake a task which you know you are not competent to do.

Extending your role

Clinical and nursing responsibilities change frequently. Similarly, your competency level may extend. If there is a question of your being required to undertake further competencies (work you are not doing now, or undertaking your present competencies in greater depth), ensure that you receive the necessary training and that your job description reflects your new "role".

It may appear clever to "have a go" at something you are not too sure about, but if a patient suffers because of your actions then *you* will be called to account.

Acceptance of gifts

It is highly unlikely that during your working life in a health care environment you will not be offered a gift of some kind, be it flowers, chocolate or money, from a client or carer.

The policy of most authorities is that staff are not permitted to accept gifts. This is in order to protect staff from any misunderstanding as to the reason for the gift being offered. For example, did the client or carer give the gift in order to receive "extra favours"? Had the patient been coerced into "offering" the gift? Or had the "gift" been taken (theft)? Some clients, in particular the elderly and the acutely ill, become disorientated and confused and can tell a different story from one day to the next.

In practice, many authorities turn a "blind eye" to the odd box of chocolates given in gratitude; but where the gift is obviously expensive or a sum of money, staff must adhere to the policy. Should you become involved, consult your supervisor and he or she will help you to explain to the client or carer why you cannot accept their kind offer. It could be suggested to the client or carer that a financial contribution to the ward or department often permits the acquisition of something which will benefit all the clients – for example, books, tapes or pictures. Any money received is sent to the relevant manager (never kept in a drawer or the drug cupboard), who in turn will write a letter of thanks and forward an official receipt.

Signing of wills

As a support worker you should avoid witnessing a client's will, however much the client insists. You should tell the client that although you would be delighted and honoured, the rules and regulations will not permit you to do this. If necessary refer the matter to your supervisor.

Disputes often arise over wills. If the dispute is in connection with whether the person was of sound mind at the time of the making of the will, or whether they were under undue influence, the only people who can be asked are the people who witnessed it. This would obviously place the support worker in a very difficult position were they asked to give an assessment some time later.

Point to remember
You may not witness the signing of a will if you are a beneficiary of it. It is best to avoid such a situation and always consult a senior colleague if in difficulty.

Making statements and attending courts

At some time during your employment you might be involved, to a lesser or greater extent, in making a report or statement of events and possibly attending court (in the case of, for example, theft or negligence). Remember what has been explained earlier about clear, concise records and writing statements of events:

- Seek advice from your supervisor or union representative.
- Do not make your statement of events from memory, but from available records.
- Do not enlarge upon what is in the records. If challenged on it you will not have anything to support your actions. *Keep it factual and accurate.*

Taking sides or trying "to please all the people all the time" will not work and may leave you open to some searching cross-examination.

If you have to give evidence in court, speak slowly and clearly, making sure you can be heard. Do not try to be a "Perry Mason" and attempt to score points! Lawyers have many "tricks of the trade" and may attempt to unnerve you. Although the lawyer has the legal expertise, you are the support worker with relevant competencies, so give your evidence accordingly.

Clients' consent

Today, **informed consent** is an important part of caring. Clients have a right to know what it is we propose to do with regard to their treatment and how we can help them.

The Patients' Charter states that every citizen has the right to be given "a clear explanation of any treatment proposed, including any risks and any alternatives", before deciding whether to agree to the treatment.

Consent forms

Invariably, medical staff will deal with the question of consent forms, explain the operation, test or treatment and obtain the client's or guardian's signature.

However, it quite often happens that a few seconds later the client asks the nearest nurse or support worker to explain in more detail what the doctor has just said. This is usually because, for a variety of reasons, the client has not fully understood and is often unwilling to ask the doctor to clarify the information.

Unless you are absolutely sure that you understand what was said and are familiar with the details of the proposed treatment, refer the matter to your supervisor.

Sensitivity in care

The fact that a client has presented to the hospital or health centre, or allowed a community nurse into their home, indicates that they are willing to accept treatment or care. This does not remove their right to have all care explained, however minor it may be. Equally, a person has the right to refuse such treatment or care if they wish.

Always explain your proposed action to the client and do not persist if the person refuses. It is possible that by persisting in your action you *could* be guilty of committing common assault.

The above guidance involves not only the care of adults, but also children. Children above all appreciate honesty, so never tell a child "this will not hurt" when you know that it will. If you explain the procedures they are more likely to cooperate.

> ### Points to remember
> - You must at all times obey the laws of the land.
> - As a member of a health care team you must be aware of your legal obligations not only to your employer but also to clients. The law does not accept that a lack of experience or knowledge is an excuse for incompetent care.
> - At all times the support worker will be expected to:
>   fulfil their legal contract
>   maintain a safe working environment
>   follow correct working procedures and policies
>   report accidents or incidents
>   communicate adequately, accurately, and above all clearly.
> - Treat people as you would wish to be treated. Clients are not there for you to practise on.

Further reading

Dewis. (1989), "Focus on COSHH – the provisions", Occupational Safety and Health, vol. 19, no. 2, pages 29–30.

Herbert. (1989), "Focus on COSHH – the practicalities", Occupational Safety and Health, vol. 19, no. 2, pages 36–38.

Finch. (1989), "Inside law – legal aspects of nursing", Nursing Standard, 29 April, pages 38–39.

Dimond. (1990), Legal Aspects of Nursing (Prentice Hall). This and the following book concentrate on the law with regard to the professional nurse, but there are many aspects which have relevance for the support worker.

Young. (1991), Law and Professional Conduct in Nursing (Scutari Press).

Practice activity
In your own area of work closely examine your actions. Do you at all times fulfil legal requirements? Discuss the points raised in this chapter with your colleagues.

11 | Caring for the dying and bereaved

Clare Fitzgibbon

‘ *To every thing there is a season, and a time to every purpose under the heaven: a time to be born, and a time to die; . . .* ’

Ecclesiastes 3: 1–2

It may seem rather strange to find a chapter on caring for the dying and the bereaved within this section on Quality. But what is quality? From Chapter 9 you will have gathered that "quality, like beauty, is in the eye of the beholder" and may mean different things to different people.

Perhaps you feel that quality of care is more relevant when the person you are caring for is going to improve in health. Then you are able to see a successful outcome of your efforts. A view frequently expressed is that the provision of care "maintains or improves quality of life", and in this connection it should always be remembered that care of the dying *is* care of the living.

The key issues of this chapter are:
■ Exploring your own feelings and fears surrounding death
■ Encouraging you to talk about death and bringing the subject right out into the open

By being able to acknowledge our own fears, feelings and emotions we hope to be one step nearer to perfecting our care of the dying and the bereaved.

The concept of death
Dr Elizabeth Kubler-Ross has said:

This chapter links with the O unit and Z3, Z4, Y2, Z8, and endorsement units Z14, Z2.

‘ *It might be helpful if more people would talk about death and dying as an intrinsic part of life just as they do not hesitate to mention if someone is expecting a new baby. . . . I am convinced that we do more harm by avoiding the issue than by using time and timing to sit, listen and share.* ’

Kubler-Ross (1970, p. 125)

We all experience emotional difficulties with the concept of death, and for care workers these difficulties are highlighted when we come into contact with people who are dying. It is understandable that many will want to turn away from the reminder that death is one of the few certainties in life and is the one thing common to us all. Death is seen by society as the final disaster, and frequently health care workers experience a sense of failure when a client dies, feeling that all their efforts have been in vain.

It is perhaps this sense of failure which has established attitudes of "distancing" or "turning away". It may also be seen as a form of self-protection in that, by avoiding involvement, you can somehow ignore your own mortality.

This attitude of distancing has perhaps been encouraged as western society has developed. The concept of death develops from early childhood and our emotional reactions to events are learned. The way grief is demonstrated, the support received from family and friends, and general reactions to death may in fact be culturally determined.

Nationally, more than 60% of deaths occur in hospital. Death has become "medicalized", which means that fewer and fewer people have witnessed a death or seen a corpse. In addition, loss of the extended family and close-knit communities has radically altered the natural cycle of birth, life and death and the way we learn to cope with life events. Rubbing shoulders with death from an early age keeps natural fear of it within limits.

It is understandable that many parents today feel the need to protect their children from such events, but this may not be the best approach.

Cultural differences

Not all cultures have developed a "medicalized" approach. There are still many societies in the world where death is embraced within the heart of the family and community. In some parts of Uganda, for example, days of feasting and drinking surround a funeral. Sorrow is present, but it is mingled with rejoicing for the life that was. Different religions have different attitudes to death, and it can be very helpful to the bereaved to have a structured ritual following the death of a loved one. Asians and Jews, to take just two examples, have a rich heritage of religious and cultural traditions. Many of these have been preserved within their communities and serve to provide great strength and comfort in times of crisis.

Point to remember
We live in a multicultural society, and although knowledge and respect for an individual's beliefs is important in all aspects of care it is particularly so when caring for the dying.

Until fairly recently the emphasis in caring for the dying was on addressing physical problems, but there has been a growing awareness of other dimensions of need and care. *Psychological*, *social* and *spiritual* aspects of care are equally important in caring for **the whole person**.

Think about
Have you ever cared for a client who was dying? If so, how did you feel when you heard that they had died? Who did you share your feelings with?

Think about
You may have experienced the death of a family member when you were young. Did you attend the funeral? Did you see your loved one following their death?

Think about
How many different cultures do you know about? Do you know about their rituals surrounding death? You could consider this as an idea for a project.

Health care workers should enquire sensitively about special needs or requirements and be aware of the appropriate person or organization to contact should this be requested.

Fear of death

Death is frequently portrayed in the media but there it appears distant, removed and therefore manageable. You can always turn off the TV or put down the newspaper or the book. However, when it comes closer to home and a family member, work colleague or neighbour dies, then death is *real*, and we then have difficulty knowing how to handle it.

There are no hard-and-fast rules in learning to cope with death. A good starting point is the ability to identify *your own* fears. This will then help you to help the dying.

Some common fears of dying and death

- Fear of suffering, of pain, of illness
- Fear of being alone, leaving loved ones behind
- Fear of "nothingness", of not existing any more
- Fear of losing control of mind or body, losing independence
- Fear of sudden death, of going to sleep
- Fear of being rejected through disfigurement, odour, or the results of deterioration
- Fear of being contagious due to AIDS.

Many such fears have been expressed by the dying. You can be of help both to the dying and their families by acknowledging and accepting these fears without being judgmental.

Sometimes you will feel helpless in the face of death. You may even see colleagues and other health care workers avoiding contact with the dying – not because they do not care, but because they do not know how to.

A great many health care workers would like to have specific do's and don'ts to follow with regard to caring for the dying. Instead, this chapter aims to provide you with a form of *toolkit*. As with any set of tools, it is the user who must select the right tool for the task and use it to its optimum capacity. The tools you need are:

Think about
Fears surrounding death are many and varied. Some may seem reasonable while others not. What are your fears?

Spend some time thinking about these and make a few notes if you wish. You may find it interesting to discuss these with a friend or colleague, who may have fears different from your own.

- communication skills
- an understanding of the stages of dying
- an understanding of feelings
- support for yourself
- consideration of moral and ethical questions.

Communication skills

As Elizabeth Kubler-Ross put it, we need "time and timing to sit, listen and share". People need to talk – not all the time, but as and when they choose. It is often at night, when the hustle and bustle of the day has passed, that the dying feel others have the time to listen. We should always have time to listen at any time of the day or night.

What would you do or say if a client asked you a question you could not answer? This is a particular fear of health care workers and often poses a dilemma. Trust is the essence of any relationship, and where you are unsure about what to say or not to say in order to avoid damaging a trusting relationship you should seek the advice and guidance of the care team or senior manager. Collaborative teamwork and effective communication will go a long way to providing consistency of care.

It is important to remain open and ready to respond appropriately. If the client says *"I'm going to die, aren't I?", you have several choices.* You might choose to say:

"Well, you are 70 and you have had a good life"
or "Oh, we will have to wait and see"
or "Don't talk like that"

or you might say:

"Do you feel like talking about it?"
or "It's not easy for you is it".

Alternatively you might say nothing and simply hold their hand.

When faced with a really difficult question, be honest with yourself and with your client and admit *"I'm not sure I'm the best person to answer it or even if I could."* Then offer to seek help from the appropriate person.

Always be guided by the client, but know the value of touch, which is often more comforting than words.

Whenever children are involved you should remember that their need for information and their understanding will depend largely on their age. Family members are generally the best people to fulfil this need, but care workers can prompt families to the needs of their children. Dying children are little different from dying adults in that many will *know* they are dying and will, if allowed, tell *you* that they are dying.

Another important aspect of communication is the language we use, particularly when talking to the bereaved. Language should be appropriate for the listener – neither full of jargon nor so simplistic as to be insulting. If the language is inappropriate or fails to provide meaning, then misunderstandings and unnecessary problems can occur.

Euphemisms surrounding death are devices we use to distance ourselves from the unthinkable, the unmentionable. Common phrases such as "lost my mother", "passed away", "kicked the bucket", "shuffled off this mortal coil" are often used in an attempt to be kind. In fact, they can be very unhelpful. To tell an elderly, distressed lady whose husband has just died that "he has gone to sleep, a long sleep" can easily create misunderstanding. Until fairly recently children were often told of a death in this way, frequently causing sleep disturbances and bedtime fears.

A common pitfall is believing that because someone close to you has died you know how it feels for someone else facing a similar loss. While such personal

Think about
How many ways can you think of to say "He has died"?

Think about
In your childhood, what words were used to explain death to you? How did you feel about the explanation? If you have ever had to explain death to a child, what words did you use?

experience will always assist in *imagining* how it feels, it *never* equips a person to say "I know how you feel". Such a comment, whilst intended sympathetically, can cause great anger in a grieving or bereaved person.

Point to remember
If you are unsure, ask a bereaved person whether they would like to be alone. Do not tell the bereaved that "time will heal", or that "death is a blessing". Remember, too, that you must accept their feelings without taking them as a personal affront.

Understanding the stages of dying

It has been through listening to the dying that a number of stages or reactions have come to be recognized. One of the best known authorities on this subject is Elizabeth Kubler-Ross, who described the dying process as: "movement through five identifiable stages, sometimes progressing sometimes transgressing, with no certainty of arrival at the final stage." These five stages are *denial*, *anger*, *bargaining*, *depression*, and *acceptance*. Such emotions are often experienced with news of *any* loss, and relatives cannot be expected to react to impending bereavement in an identical manner.

Think about
To help you understand the stages of dying and the feelings and emotions aroused, consider how you felt about the material loss of something of value to you – for example, an item of jewellery, your wallet, your car. Should you suffer a major loss in terms of material possessions, it may mean that your way of life alters radically, and your reactions to such a loss can be compared in all but their intensity and the depth of the emotion involved to the reactions experienced when we lose a loved one.

It is worth looking at the five stages in some detail, thinking of them as milestones along a journey, some of which will be seen and recognized while others may be missed. If you consider dying as a journey, then think of it as one with many routes, some of which will be crowded with emotions.

Denial: "No, not me"
This is the initial phase most often displayed by clients and families in their refusal to accept the reality of impending death. It would seem that the brain can refuse to accept any information which appears to be unthinkable and impossible. If we deny it, perhaps it will go away. Perhaps it hasn't really happened. Most people will move on from this stage, but a few will outwardly cling to denial as a way of coping.

Point to remember
If outright denial is to be challenged, then it must be done gently by someone expert in counselling skills.

Anger: "Why me? Why now?"

Anger is often used as a disguise for underlying fears and anxieties. Wherever anger is directed, it can usually be defused if carers can accept it without taking it as a personal criticism or affront. Time is needed to understand the feelings being expressed.

Bargaining: "Yes, it is happening; but if . . . "

In this stage there is an attempt to bargain with doctors or with God for some remission or cure. The client or relatives may seek other opinions or other forms of treatment. Professional carers must avoid being judgmental but must be supportive and prepared to provide all necessary information to enable individuals to arrive at an informed decision which is not harmful.

Depression

Depression is closely associated with actual or anticipated loss. Sadness that life will end is felt by almost everyone facing death and may cause the individual to be withdrawn and submissive. However, if the depression is explored there may be underlying causes which, with support, can be dealt with and in some cases treatment offered and the condition alleviated.

Acceptance

There are many degrees of acceptance.

Active acceptance is completely different from passive resignation: the former brings something positive and vital to the client while the latter, being essentially negative, casts a shadow of gloom across the final phase of the client's illness.
Twycross (1983)

Not everyone will reach this stage, and of those who have there may be a feeling of betrayal of their loved ones: "as if I'm giving up". Relatives may also experience this sentiment. It is important to remember that while relatives also travel this road they may reach different milestones at different times.

Example

Sarah was 18 when she learnt that she was dying. Many weeks before her death she reached the stage of acceptance, and at this point she decided to put everything in order. She wrote letters, distributed her possessions and planned her own funeral. Her family were not at the same stage in the journey and they found this behaviour exceedingly distressing.

In such a situation a **Macmillan nurse** or member of the care team can assist both parties to understand each other's feelings, emotions and difficulties.

Throughout all these stages perhaps the most important thing to consider is

> **Think about**
> Think about your lost item of value. Did you feel anger? Were you angry at yourself or angry with others, or both?

hope. For far too many people – including some professional carers – involvement in the process of dying creates a feeling of hopelessness. Yet hope is the one thing that can coexist throughout the whole journey.

In recognizing that the status of dying is more readily acknowledged in those with a terminal illness, we should be aware that death can occur at any time in any area of care.

❝If we are to raise the status of the care of the elderly in the same way as the Hospice movement has raised the status of cancer care, we may need to recognise that we are all at different stages on the road to death, with some nearer than others. The care of the elderly IS the care of the dying, just as it is the care of the living.❞

Clive Seale (1993)

Equally, we need to recognize the special needs of the many who die as a result of trauma, accident or heart attack, where the journey may be one of only hours or days. Hope for this last group will be different from that of the elderly or terminally ill. Right up to the moment of death there can be active treatment and hope of recovery.

Hope for the elderly or terminally ill has shifted from one of recovery or cure to one of comfort. Even here, there are those who need to hope for something unforeseen in the form of a cure or miracle. This hope should not be destroyed.

Perhaps in this situation hope is more about realistic goal setting, about being able to listen to a favourite piece of music, about the pleasure of a warm bath or – as one gentleman said – "just waking up to another day".

Understanding feelings

Feelings in normal grief closely reflect those described in the stages of dying.

■ **Shock and disbelief**. These most often occur in cases of sudden death but can arise even when death has been expected. Sometimes this is accompanied by physical symptoms of pallor, sweating and palpitations.

■ **Numbness** – being unable to feel anything. As in denial, the brain can refuse to accept information. This numbness can last for up to two or more weeks.

■ **Anger**. This can be directed at the professionals who could not prevent the death, or at the dead person for leaving.

■ **Sadness**. This is a sadness for the life that has gone, for the lost future.

■ **Guilt**. This feeling can often be irrational. The bereaved person may feel that they did not do enough or that it was due to them that the person died.

Practice point
Consider ideas for realistic goal setting as ways of maintaining hope with a dying client.

■ **Relief** – particularly when the loved-one has suffered. Even relief can be tempered with guilt at being the one who is still alive.

■ **Anxiety** – fear of coping alone.

■ **Fatigue** – often unexpected and closely related to apathy and listlessness.

■ **Yearning**. Pining for the one who has died is common amongst bereaved persons.

■ **Searching** – for the familiar face in a crowd, hearing his/her voice.

■ **Loneliness** – especially in those who have lost a partner.

■ **Emancipation**. This sense of freedom can seem to be inappropriate but can be real for someone who has been subject to abuse or ill-treatment.

All these feelings may be jumbled up. As with the stages of dying, they do not come in any prescribed order. You must learn to recognize and be sensitive to these feelings and emotions.

Support for yourself

It seems appropriate at this point to consider how you can cope with the many emotions you will experience in your care of the dying and the bereaved. This quotation from Sheila Cassidy will bring to many of you an echo of your own feelings:

‘*At heart, professional loving is about competence, empathy and communication. It is about becoming sensitive to the pain of others and therefore terribly vulnerable. For me, as for many, it is a way of caring which I aspire to, but achieve only some of the time. It is a costly loving for which I am repaid a hundred fold.*’

Cassidy (1988)

Although professional carers working specifically with the dying have developed specialist skills, anybody who has a caring role can learn not only from the specialists such as the Macmillan nurse or **hospice** staff, but also from the dying themselves.

Just as the stages and feelings of the dying and bereaved will vary enormously, so too will yours. Facing the grief of others can release powerful unexpressed emotions of your own. It is important to understand the following:

■ Wherever you work you are not in isolation but are a member of a whole team.

■ Sharing and supporting amongst team members is essential.

■ Sharing the shedding of tears in the presence of a client or relative is *not* unprofessional.

■ Remember that your presence alone, in silence, can be a comfort.

> **Think about**
> No man is an island and within your area of work you will have some form of support network. Think about the support network you have and how you might, if necessary, improve it.

Consideration of moral and ethical questions

In order to "relieve distress" there is much we need to consider, not least that of **ethics** or **moral questions** which may affect you.

Most people, when asked about ethics in caring, will cite the big dilemmas of abortion, euthanasia, truth-telling and compulsory psychiatric treatment – and this is to a large extent understandable because these focus upon the feelings and beliefs of individuals and their ideas of right and wrong.

It is important to be able to examine your own feelings and attitudes. How you value life, death and health, your faith and your thoughts on the meaning of life will all have an effect on your physical and emotional care of your client. Each and every one of us carries with us our own "collection" of personal feelings about most major life issues. This collection of feelings or values will be reflected in the care we give.

With this in mind it is important not to be judgmental in care situations. It is not your feelings that are important. What is important is that the wishes of the client and the family can be met by being kept fully informed of the choices and services available to them. In that way, it is hoped, wishes can be met – *not our wishes as health care workers and what we believe to be right*, but the wishes of the dying person and the family and what *they* most want.

Think about

When a moral conflict occurs within yourself, how do you deal with it? Consider, for example, that a young man has attempted suicide by taking an overdose of a drug. The treatment required to save his life is very expensive in terms of time, money and care and has a slim chance of success. Would you feel angry about the amount of effort being made to save his life? Would this affect the way in which you provided care to this individual?

Now consider that an elderly woman is in severe pain from terminal cancer. She has overdosed on a drug. Would you feel or act differently in this case? If so, why? If not, why not?

Who or where would you go to for support, guidance and advice? Wherever or whenever you do face such a conflict, it is important that you are able to discuss it with the most appropriate person, who will usually be your supervisor or manager. Where your feelings and beliefs come into conflict with your care, you must acknowledge this to avoid discriminating, making assumptions or judgments about an individual.

In caring for the dying and bereaved we place ourselves alongside those who suffer. Such suffering touches us at a deep and powerful level, stirs our capacity to love and reaches us at the level of our common destiny.

A "Bill of Rights"

Wherever you work remember your client's rights. Discuss these with your colleagues. How can you ensure that you fully understand these rights? How can you ensure that these rights will be upheld? The following "Bill of Rights" may help you consider these issues further. It was drawn up by Amelia Barbus and is cited by Elizabeth Kubler-Ross in *Dealing with Death and Dying* (1984).

The dying client's Bill of Rights

- I have the right to be treated as a living human being until I die.
- I have the right to maintain a sense of hopefulness, however changing its focus might be.
- I have the right to be cared for by those who can maintain a sense of hopefulness, however changing this might be.
- I have the right to express my feelings and emotions about my approaching death in my own way.
- I have the right to participate in decisions concerning my care.
- I have the right to expect continuing medical and nursing attention, even though "cure" goals must be changed to "comfort" goals.
- I have the right not to die alone.
- I have the right to be free of pain.
- I have the right to have my questions answered honestly.
- I have the right not to be deceived.
- I have the right to have help from and for my family in accepting my death.
- I have the right to die in peace and dignity.
- I have the right to retain my individuality and not be judged for my decisions that may be contrary to the beliefs of others.
- I have the right to discuss and enlarge my religious and/or spiritual experiences, whatever these may mean to others.
- I have the right to expect that the sanctity of the human body will be respected after death.
- I have the right to be cared for by caring, sensitive, knowledgeable people who will attempt to understand my needs and will be able to gain some satisfaction in helping me face my death.

Points to remember

- Learning to cope with death and dying is not easy and will be a stressful learning process – but the most worthwhile is not always the easiest.
- Be aware of your own fears and feelings and be sensitive to the fears and feelings of others.
- Respect for people is paramount in caring.
- Care for clients without being judgmental.
- Remember that you are not alone, and if in doubt always ask.

Glossary

Distancing. In this context, a mental barrier is set up between the carer and the person dying – usually to avoid acknowledging one's own fears and feelings.

Euphemism. Use of a pleasanter, less direct word for something unpleasant.

Macmillan nurse. The Macmillan nurse is a specialist who usually works with people who have cancer. The funding for the specialist nurse always arises initially from the Cancer Relief Macmillan Fund, a national charitable organization.

Hospice movement. Originally, a medieval guest house or way station for pilgrims and travellers; currently used to designate either a place or a philosophy of care for persons in the last stages of life and their families. The concept of a hospice is that of a caring community of professional and non-professional people, supplemented by volunteer services.

Further reading

Green. (1991), Death with Dignity (Nursing Times Publications). Meeting the spiritual needs of clients in a multi cultural society.

Kubler-Ross. (1984), Dealing with Death and Dying, 2nd edn (Springhouse Corporation). Dr Elizabeth Kubler-Ross is a well-known author on the subject of death and dying. This book offers advice on how to deal with the feelings and fears of the client, the family and yourself.

Buckman. (1988), I Don't Know What to Say (Macmillan). Deals with the subject of death in an honest, open and caring way. Also provides information on how to help and support someone who is dying.

Dickenson and Johnson. (eds) (1993), Death, Dying and Bereavement (Sage/Open University). This book will be of interest to all concerned with the issues surrounding death, and in particular to those directly involved in the support of the dying or bereaved people, whether as paid carers, family members, friends or volunteers.

REFERENCES

Cassidy S. (1988). *Sharing the Darkness* (Darton, Longman and Todd).

Kubler-Ross E. (1970). *On Death and Dying* (Tavistock).

Seale C. (1993). "Demographic change and the care of the dying", in Dickenson D. and Johnson M. (eds), *Death, Dying and Bereavement* (Sage/Open University).

Twycross R.G. (1983). *The Dying Patient* (CMF Publications).

Practice activity
There are a number of hospices throughout the country. Try to arrange a visit to one near you and spend some time with the staff and the clients. Alternatively or in addition, contact your local Macmillan nursing service and arrange to meet with one of the nurses.

Controlling infection in health care settings

12

Rozila Horton

Every individual, be it in their own home, a health care setting or a social environment, will have encountered at least one episode of infection. Many germs (organisms) can be found in and around the human body at all times, usually living in perfect harmony with humans. When infection occurs this usually means that the conditions are favourable for the organisms to grow and multiply sufficiently to overwhelm the body's defences. There are also situations where the body's defences are damaged and unable to resist the organisms. This may be due to a condition present from birth, a disease of the immune system itself, or because of certain treatments which damage the body's mechanism.

The subject of infection control is vast, dealing with many complexities such as how the human body protects itself and what factors interfere with the body's ability to fight diseases. The aspect which is important here is the responsibility that health care workers have for reducing the risk of infection to clients under their care and to themselves.

Many sick and vulnerable people are congregated within a care setting and this provides an ideal opportunity for organisms to cause infection and for that infection to be transmitted to others. Many practices which are designed to help the client can, inadvertently, result in infection. Infecting organisms can be transferred from an infected source either on care giver's hands or by use of a contaminated item of equipment on a non-infected person. Since infection-producing organisms may be encountered any-where, staff should be aware not only of the factors which contribute to the spread of infection, but also how to prevent or minimize the risk of infection to those under their care, as well as to protect themselves.

By virtue of the knowledge gained as a care giver, opportunities for guiding and educating clients should not be missed. Today there is much emphasis on empowering clients to participate and have a say in their own care. These possibilities present themselves in health care settings as well as in clients' own homes when carrying out domiciliary visits.

This chapter links with units O, U4, U5 and endorsement unit U3.

The key issues of this chapter are:
- What we mean by infection
- Immunity and the human body
- The effect infections have on the individual as well as on the organization
- The chain of infection
- The basis of safe practice
- A safe environment
- Safe care practices
- Infection control in client's own home
- Patterns of infection

What is meant by infection?

The term "infection" is used when **pathogenic** (disease producing) organisms have entered the body, invaded the body tissue, multiplied and produced a response. This may be shown as inflammation following a cut or surrounding a cannula site, or as pus in a surgical wound. Alternatively, the whole body may be affected as in childhood infections (e.g. measles and chickenpox).

The period of time between the organism entering the body and the appearance of signs and symptoms is referred to as the "**incubation period**". This can range from hours to several days or, in some instances as in "human immunodeficiency virus" (HIV), many years. This period is specific to each disease.

Many of the symptoms of disease – for example fever, headache, nausea – are caused by the **toxins** produced by the organism. The toxins enter the bloodstream and travel round the body targeting specific cells and organs. Where there is a localized rapid increase in the number of organisms, some body tissue is destroyed with the resulting formation of pus.

Organisms may be so small that they can only be seen with the help of a microscope; these are known as "micro-organisms". Some organisms, such as worms, are large enough to be visible to the eye (Hare and Cooke 1984). Not all organisms cause disease, but we shall now consider some that may.

- **Bacteria** are single cells and are classified according to their shape, which may be spherical, rod-shaped or spiral. Many bacteria live on and within the human body and these are called "resident" or "endogenous" organisms. They are not usually harmful and may even help protect the individual. In certain circumstances these organisms become pathogenic and cause disease, or take the opportunity in a susceptible person to set up an infectious process. Bacteria are the major cause of disease.
- **Viruses** are the smallest of the pathogenic organisms and cause disease by entering the cells of the body. There are many varieties and strains of viruses, which makes treatment and control very difficult. The common cold is due to a virus.

- **Fungi** exist either as oval, yeast-like structures or as mycelial threads which produce spores.
- **Protozoa** are single-celled organisms which belong to the animal kingdom. Diseases that are caused by protozoa include malaria and sleeping sickness.
- **Worms** are often found as parasites in humans and animals. Most worm infections are transmitted from person to person via food and water which has been contaminated by faeces.

Micro-organisms which live in or on human bodies are known as "resident" organisms. Organisms of most concern are those known as "transient" which cause infection by being transferred on hands of carers and the equipment they use. This is called "cross infection".

For an infection to occur, a number of factors have to be present. These include the organism causing the disease, the place it lives and the method by which the micro-organism is transmitted to the susceptible person. These are discussed later.

Patterns of infection

- *Individual* – People acquire similar infections without having been in contact with each other. These are known as "sporadic infections" because they occur as isolated incidents.
- *Endemic* – Different countries throughout the world have their own level of infection which remains constant within their own population. Diseases such as measles, chickenpox and mumps may be more prevalent in some countries than in others.
- *Epidemic* – Unlike endemic infection which remains at a constant level, epidemic infection can either be an unexpected increase in the level of endemic infection or an outbreak.

Immunity and the human body

How does our body protect us from infection, and why? When a person has been in contact with an infected person, why have they not always contracted the disease? Infectious diseases *appear* to be selective, but in fact it is not the organism which is selective but the ability of the body to protect itself by the mechanism known as **immunity**.

Nature has provided humans with an array of cells which identify harmful organisms and have the ability to fight them. These include non-specific mechanisms like the skin and secretory linings of the respiratory, gastrointestinal and urogenital tracts. Intact skin acts as a first line of defence, but skin and body secretions act as both physical and chemical barriers.

Specific cells in the blood and lymphatic systems are programmed to fight foreign invading organisms, which are usually called **antigens**. These specific cells are called **T** and **B** cells. The T cells can kill antigens directly and recognize

Think about
Think about a group of people with whom you work, colleagues and clients. Have you noticed that sometimes a common cold will affect everyone, while at other times only one person will be affected?

the difference between those cells which belong to the body and those which do not.

The T cells also act as instructors to the B cells, prompting the B cells to respond. The B cells are responsible for the production of **antibodies**. Each antibody is designed to attack a specific disease. For example, when a person contracts measles the B cells will manufacture antibodies against the measles virus. Should that person come in contact with the measles virus again, the B cells remember and rapidly produce antibodies from the original template. This will affect the **virulence** of the attack. Symptoms of the virus infection will either be unnoticeable or reduced.

This mechanism is effective with a wide range of infectious diseases, but there are some exceptions, notably HIV. The degree and timed protection provided by the "immune response" varies widely from one organism to another. Protection against the common cold is short-lived, whereas protection against measles is for life. Figure 12.1 illustrates the immune response to infection.

Methods of assisting the immune response

Through scientific discoveries and an increasing knowledge of the body, methods of assisting the immune response have been developed. Two of these methods are described as **passive** and **active immunity**.

Passive immunity

At birth the immune system is not fully developed, but nature provides a degree of protection for the newborn. During fetal growth and development, the antibodies which the mother has produced are passed to the baby via the placenta. This provides protection for the baby, *but only to infections to which the mother has been exposed.*

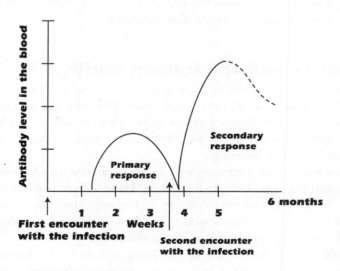

Figure 12.1   Immune response to infection

Another method of transferring antibodies from mother to baby is through breast milk, which is an important reason for encouraging breast-feeding. The antibodies in the breast milk will protect the baby for up to 6 months, after which the baby's immune system will be sufficiently mature to produce its own defences.

In a similar way, passive immunity can be given to adults. This is given in the form of an injection or serum which contains specific antibodies. This method can be used to protect people travelling to countries where specific diseases are endemic; but as in the newborn, the protection offered by passive immunity lasts only a very short time, probably not more than 6 months.

Active immunity

Active immunization means that there has been a stimulation of the immune system either through contracting the disease, or by artificially stimulating the body to respond to the disease. It is known that, following recovery from infections such as measles and whooping cough, the person becomes immune to the organism and is not likely to suffer a second attack. The obvious disadvantage of this method of obtaining immunity is that it can be acquired only by having an attack of the disease. As many infectious diseases can be fatal, or produce serious side-effects, this is not the most desirable way of achieving immunity. However, **vaccination** with carefully prepared specific organisms can stimulate the body's immune system, to respond in the same way without having to suffer an attack of the disease.

Vaccines are prepared in a number of ways – from live but weakened organisms as in measles, mumps and rubella, to dead organisms as in whooping cough and typhoid vaccine.

Table 12.1 A recommended immunization programme for children

Vaccine	Age	Notes
DTP and polio	2 months	1st dose
	3 months	2nd dose
	4 months	3rd dose
MMR	12–18 months	Can be given at any age over 12 months
Booster DT and polio	4–5 years	
Rubella	10–14 years	Girls only
BCG	10–14 years or infancy	Interval of 3 weeks between BCG and rubella
Booster tetanus and polio	15–18 years	

DTP = diphtheria/tetanus/whooping cough (pertussis); MMR = measles/mumps/rubella; BCG = tuberculosis vaccine; polio = poliomyelitis.

Active immunization can provide lifelong protection, although some organisms (e.g. tetanus) will require reactivation in the form of a "booster" at certain intervals.

Immunization programmes

The development of artificially induced active immunity for certain diseases has had a major impact throughout the world. Smallpox has been completely wiped out and the incidence of poliomyelitis has decreased dramatically.

Immunization programmes are recommended for all infants and children, and they usually begin when the child is 2–3 months old. Table 12.1 shows a typical immunization programme (DoH 1992), but this schedule may differ in other countries.

Children should therefore have received the following vaccines:

- by 6 months – three doses of DTP and polio, or DT and polio
- by 18 months – measles/mumps/rubella
- by school entry – fourth DT and polio; MMR if missed earlier
- between 10 and 14 years – BCG; rubella for girls
- before leaving school – fifth polio and tetanus.

Adults should receive the following vaccines:

- women seronegative for rubella – rubella
- previously unimmunized individuals – polio, tetanus
- individuals in high-risk groups – hepatitis B, influenza.

In the UK, some diseases are **notifiable** by law to the Consultant in Communicable Disease Control (CCDC). Examples are measles, whooping cough and tuberculosis. The World Health Organization (WHO) monitors outbreaks of infectious diseases throughout the world, and where necessary initiates appropriate preventative and control measures.

Health education and promotion

As a support worker you have a vital role in health education and health promotion, and immunization is an important preventative measure designed to improve the nation's health and to reduce morbidity and mortality. Many people today have become complacent and are unaware of the horrors of diseases such as poliomyelitis and diphtheria.

Health education is necessary to encourage the public to take up the immunization programmes offered, but it must also be recognized that individuals have a right to refuse immunization. Some vaccinations may produce mild symptoms such as low-grade pyrexia (fever) and a general feeling of being unwell, but these symptoms usually last only a short time. On very rare occasions an **allergic reaction** may occur which can range from mild to severe symptoms, as in anaphylaxis. To put this risk into perspective, 25 million people were immunized between 1978 and 1989 in the UK, with only 118 anaphylactic reactions. No deaths were reported from the subsequent anaphylaxis during this period (DoH 1992).

The development of vaccines against specific diseases has undoubtedly created a safer environment for everyone, but the spectrum of infectious agents changes not only with the passage of time but also with the introduction of drugs and chemicals designed to destroy them. Not all infections can be eradicated by drugs or chemicals. Indeed, with the widespread use of antibiotics over the past 60 years, many organisms have been able to develop a **resistance** to a number of drugs. So, "prevention is better than cure".

The next part of the chapter considers the effect infection has upon individuals and organizations, and most importantly the measures which can be taken to control and reduce the spread of infection.

The effect of infection in hospitals

It is estimated that up to 20% of clients in acute hospitals may be infected at any given time. Not all of these infections have occurred whilst in hospital. In fact, about half of these clients are already infected or are incubating the disease when they are admitted.

Carers have very little control over these **community-acquired infections** (CAI) but need to appreciate that they may be transmitted to other susceptible clients and to care staff. The remaining 10% of infected clients have developed their infection 48 hours after entering a hospital, so these are called **hospital-acquired infections** (HAI) or "nosocomial" infections.

This does not necessarily mean that the infection occurred as a direct result of practices or treatment – it means simply that it occurred during hospitalization. The source of the infection may be the organisms already present in or on the body, another client or a member of staff already infected who is carrying the disease, or it may be a result of nursing practice and/or treatment.

Infections carry with them costs to both the client and the hospital. Infected clients have to stay in hospital longer (on an average four more days than non-infected clients), thus leading to a possible loss of earnings for them. Pain associated with infection can lead to loss of or reduced physical function, and many infections prove fatal (Ayliffe, Collins and Taylor 1990). Hospital-acquired infections were said to cost the National Health Service £117 million in 1987, and the cost of caring is rising daily.

Infected clients require additional investigations, drugs, dressings, therapies and added nursing and medical time. As funding now follows the client, increased length of stay due to infection affects the incoming finances as well as increasing the waiting lists of the hospital.

It has been suggested that a third of all infections may be prevented. Since such prevention could save many millions of pounds, it is essential to consider the cost of infections not only to the client but also to the organization. All health care workers have a role to play in infection control, but bedside care-givers carry by far the biggest responsibility for the protection of their clients, their relatives and themselves. This requires an understanding of all the different factors which

Think about
Can you estimate how many clients entering your health care setting will have an infection already present?

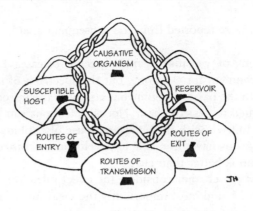

Figure 12.2   The chain of infection

lead to infection and the steps which may be taken to reduce the risk of infection to both clients and carers.

The chain of infection

Humans and micro-organisms normally live in harmony, but Figure 12.2 shows components which come together when infection develops.

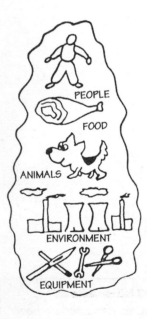

- **Causative organisms** are those capable of causing the infection. We have seen that these may be bacteria, viruses or fungi.
- **Reservoirs** are the places or sources where these organisms live and where they may or may not multiply. The sources can be people, food, animals, the environment or equipment. Clients and health care personnel may be suffering from infections or may be carrying the organism which may not show up as symptoms of infection in themselves but can cause infections in others if transmitted.
- **Routes of exit** are points in humans and animals whence these organisms may leave the body, such as skin and mucous membranes, blood, or the respiratory, gastrointestinal and genitourinary tracts.
- **Routes of transmission** are the methods by which the infectious organism is transferred from its reservoir to the susceptible person. **Direct contact** may be person-to-person spread or a person coming into direct contact with the source of infection (e.g. faeces in faecal oral transmission). **Indirect contact** is when a contaminated piece of equipment is used. Spread may be **air-borne**, through dust particles. It may be **vector-borne**, which is transmission by flies, mosquitoes etc. Another example is food poisoning affecting all those eating the same food.
- **Routes of entry** are identical to routes of exit. For example, infection can enter the body through the skin, when siting a cannula, through a sharps injury, or by catheterization through the genitourinary tract.
- **A susceptible host** is a person who is lacking in the ability to resist the

harmful or pathogenic effects of organisms. Many factors result in a lowered resistance to infection. The very young and the very old are less able to fight infection, as are those who suffer from diabetes or circulatory or respiratory problems. Many clients enter a hospital because they have a condition which has already interfered with their immune system or because they are given drugs and therapies which depress those body cells designed to help fight infection. In hospitals they may be given an intravenous infusion, feeding and breathing tubes which all bypass their normal defence mechanisms. Because of these factors, organisms not normally associated with infection may take advantage of the lowered resistance of the body. Infections resulting from this are said to be **opportunistic**.

Last but not least, the activities of care givers which are designed to *help* clients may actually pose a risk of infection. Effective infection control means becoming a safe practitioner by being aware of the hazards associated with procedures and by knowing how to eliminate these risks, as well as ensuring that care givers themselves are protected. The danger lies not only in the fact that the carer may become infected, but also that the carer risks transmitting the organism or infection to all those coming in contact with them.

The basics of safe practice

In most health care settings, a set of policies and protocols is implemented designed to protect staff, clients and the organization. It is imperative that all health care personnel familiarize themselves with those that directly affect their own area of work.

Employee health

Each health care employer should have a programme for screening staff on employment, for providing appropriate immunization, and for dealing with accidents such as sharps and needlestick injuries from used sharp objects and needles. Individual members of staff also carry a personal accountability and responsibility for protecting themselves as well as others by reporting incidents and exposures.

Point to remember

Many instances of diarrhoea in staff go unreported, resulting in transmission to other staff and/or clients and thus causing an outbreak of infection. Diarrhoea can be devastating for people already compromised by illness or injury.

A safe environment

Environmental safety involves all the fixtures, fittings, supplies and services, and includes clients, staff and visitors. It also involves waste and other materials

Think about

Can you think of care practices which could help prevent the spread of micro-organisms?

Practice point

▶ What responsibility do you have as an employee, for protecting those in your care?

▶ Do you know if there are standards, procedures or protocols for infection control where you work?

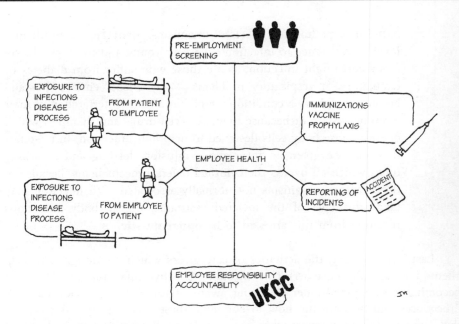

Figure 12.3 Employee health

which are removed from the care environment. Everyone working in a health care setting, therefore, carries either a direct or indirect responsibility for protecting clients, staff and visitors.

In a hospital setting, engineers play a vital role in maintaining equipment

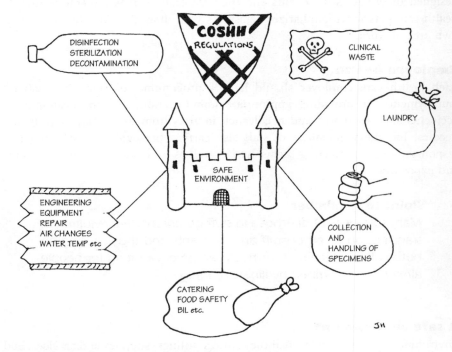

Figure 12.4 Factors in the safe environment

and items so that end-products (e.g. sterile items, water sprays from the air conditioning system or bedpans being processed in a washer) are safe for people coming in contact with them. Even the hot water has to be kept at the correct temperature so that organisms such as legionella do not flourish in water storage tanks.

All members of the catering staff have a specific responsibility for ensuring that the food served to clients, staff and visitors is safe. In fact anyone who handles food needs to be aware of food safety regulations.

Clinical waste and used linen can pose a risk to the personnel at the point where they are generated and/or where these are processed. The guidelines on safe disposal of waste and management of linen with the accompanying colour-coding system of bags (see later) are designed to eliminate or minimize such risks.

The responsibility for correct disposal rests with each carer. Careless disposal of a used needle or a sharp instrument can put other colleagues at risk.

Waste disposal facilities in community settings may be different from that in hospitals. Care staff need to familiarize themselves with the arrangements which are agreed with the local authority. In the majority of instances used linen can be safely washed in a domestic washing machine.

There are specific protocols which have to be followed in cases of needlestick or sharps injuries from used items. It is vitally important that such injuries are *reported* to the appropriate authority and that local procedures for "sharps injury", are followed.

Safe client care practice

The best method for the protection of clients is to ensure that all care activities are safe. Some simple but effective practices are discussed below.

Handwashing

Hands are used to comfort and heal as well as to minister physical needs. The client may or may not have an infection, but in carrying out these functions hands come in contact with the client's body, body secretions and excretions as well as with contaminated linen and waste.

It is of paramount importance that hands are washed to remove transient organisms. Organisms cannot be seen with the naked eye but may be picked up when carrying out most client care activities and procedures. Most organizations now advise the use of disposable gloves when dealing with body excretions and secretions to protect the care giver, but hands still need to be washed on completing the activity. Correct handwashing technique is necessary to ensure that all areas of hands are washed. Thorough rinsing and drying of hands is necessary to prevent skin problems.

Practice point
Do you know the rationale for the colour-coded bags in your own organization? What steps should you follow in instances of sharps injury?

Think about
Many micro-organisms are happily resident on our body. We cannot get rid of them completely nor should we try, since we need them. Therefore, consider what it is that you are trying to remove during normal social handwash after direct contact with a client or a used piece of equipment?

> **Practice point**
> **Hands should be washed before**:
>   caring for a susceptible client
>   preparing or handling food
>   leaving working areas (e.g. before going to lavatory, canteen or going home)
>   contact with clients in intensive care units (ICU) or special care baby units (SCBU).
>
> **Hands should be washed after**:
>   dealing with body fluids, excretions or secretions (gloves are recommended in this situation)
>   touching urine measuring devices, suction bottles, sputum collecting pots etc.
>   caring for clients who are infected or colonized
>   using toilet, blowing or touching one's nose
>   contact with clients in ICU or SCBU.
>
> Soap and water are sufficient to remove transient organisms.
> In areas where clients are vulnerable even to low pathogenic resident organisms, an antiseptic-based handwash or handrub is desirable.

Bedmaking

Clients who are infected or colonized with many harmful organisms may shed these from their body on to the bedding. Shaking of bedclothes is inadvisable since these organisms would be dispersed into the atmosphere. Since the floor is likely to be contaminated with these organisms settling there, it is important that bedclothes do not touch the floor during bedmaking. This will stop organisms from the floor being transferred to the bed.

Bedbathing

Clients may have organisms on the skin which can be picked up on the washcloth during bedbathing and transferred from one part of the body to another. Water must be changed at least once during bedbathing and washcloths rinsed thoroughly under running hot water after use and left to dry. Washbowls can also harbour organisms. They should be washed and dried thoroughly after each use and stored inverted.

During bedmaking, bedbathing, washing and turning clients who are incontinent, there may be a possibility of the uniform becoming contaminated and the use of plastic aprons is recommended when undertaking these procedures.

> **Point to remember**
> Many care givers will be required to empty urinary catheter bags. Organisms can ascend from the tap to the bladder and cause infection. Using disposable gloves and a clean dry receptacle for emptying the catheter bag is the recommended practice. Plastic aprons are advisable to prevent contamination of

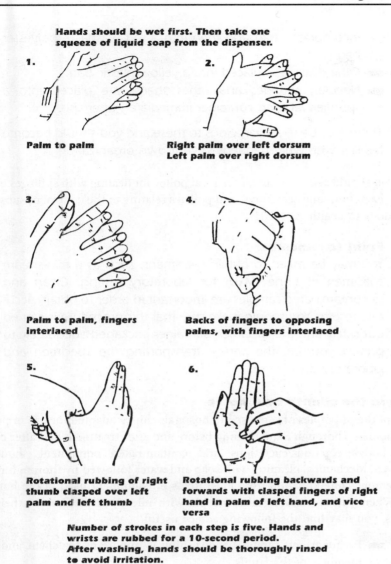

Hands should be wet first. Then take one squeeze of liquid soap from the dispenser.

1.

2.

Palm to palm

**Right palm over left dorsum
Left palm over right dorsum**

3.

4.

Palm to palm, fingers interlaced

Backs of fingers to opposing palms, with fingers interlaced

5.

6.

Rotational rubbing of right thumb clasped over left palm and left thumb

Rotational rubbing backwards and forwards with clasped fingers of right hand in palm of left hand, and vice versa

**Number of strokes in each step is five. Hands and wrists are rubbed for a 10-second period.
After washing, hands should be thoroughly rinsed to avoid irritation.**

Figure 12.5   Handwashing technique

your uniform from splashes of urine during the emptying procedure. The receptacle should be washed, rinsed and stored inverted to dry thoroughly between use. Hands should be washed on removing gloves.

Disposal of linen and waste

Hospitals in the UK operate a colour-coding system of bags of linen and waste.

Example

■ Soiled and fouled linen is placed in a white nylon bag.
■ Infected linen is placed in a biodegradable or an alginate-

incorporated bag and then into a red washable polyester bag.
- Clinical waste is placed into a yellow plastic bag.
- Needles, syringes and other sharps are placed into a specified labelled container immediately after use.

There may be slight variations to these and you should become familiar with what happens in your own organization.

You should also be aware of the local policy for dealing with spillages of body fluids, excretions and secretions, and policies relating to the control of substances hazardous to health (COSHH).

Point to remember
You may be asked to obtain specimens, such as a mid-stream specimen of urine (MSU) for laboratory testing. Clean and uncontaminated samples are important in order to obtain accurate results. You should make sure that this procedure is carried out safely and the specimen container packaged adequately to protect yourself, the person transporting the specimen and laboratory staff.

Care in the client's own home

Most of the principles of care used in hospitals can be adapted for use in people's own homes. Thorough handwashing before and after treatment and after contact with body secretions/excretions and contaminated equipment should be followed. Mechanical cleaning with soap and water followed by thorough rinsing will remove contamination from most items of equipment used in the home.

When you are looking after people with infectious diseases in their own homes, you may find the following advice useful.

- Frequent and careful handwashing is important for client and other members of the family.
- Handwash before handling food and utensils when preparing food.
- Crockery and cutlery must be washed in a dishwasher or in very hot water.
- Items of clothing from infected clients may be washed in the domestic washing machine using the hot wash cycle.

It is important to remember that family members who are newborn, elderly or diabetic, or have cancer or suffer from an immunosuppressive disease, are particularly susceptible to infection.

Current infection control problems

In your working situation you are likely to encounter clients with a variety of infections where particular care/practice have to be considered. To allow for individual care to be given, the following points should be thought about:

- what the infection is
- which part of the body is infected
- how it may be transmitted
- measures taken to stop spread
- the treatment prescribed
- when precautions should be discontinued.

Think about
Think of a client you have nursed recently with an infection which was resistant to a number of antibiotics. What precautions were you asked to take and why?

For yourself you need to consider all the above points plus your own values, attitude and beliefs about the specific infection and how it affects the client. It is also useful to remember the effect of isolation nursing upon the client and relatives.

As a carer you are likely to come across several infections. Only one or two examples are given here – there are many more. Appropriate advice is always available from colleagues, the Infection Control Nurse and in Infection Control Policy manuals. It is important that you know the rationale for the practice you are asked to carry out and you have peace of mind. If unsure, consult the above-mentioned people.

Clients who are infected or colonized with antibiotic-resistant organisms

Today clients are treated with a wide range of antibiotics both in the community and in hospitals. This has resulted in organisms developing resistance to the very antibiotics designed to cure them. The scope for treatment for these clients becomes very limited, which may lead to serious morbidity or even death.

Remember that these resistant organisms can spread easily from one client to another on hands of the care staff and via used equipment.

Meningitis

The linings (membranes) of the brain or spinal cord are inflamed. Many different microorganisms and conditions are associated with this disease. The young and the old tend to be affected, but the infection can be seen in all age groups. Most cases of meningitis are sporadic, although current guidelines recommend that some close contacts of the infected client should be prescribed antibiotics to prevent disease in them. Such **prophylaxis** is not usually required in care staff.

These clients are usually isolated to ensure quiet surroundings. Elaborate precautions are rarely required, although some cases of meningitis are accompanied by a skin rash which may be infectious. Plastic aprons and gloves and careful handwashing are advised.

Meningitis creates anxiety in relatives and friends of the client. They require much support and reassurance which you can give provided you have a basic understanding of the condition.

Diarrhoeal illness

This is a common occurrence in health care settings. Both staff and clients may be affected. Many organisms can cause this illness but the most common causes are viruses. The symptoms are usually of short duration, but the spread can be rapid through a group of susceptible people. Some diarrhoeal diseases result from the use of antibiotics. Cross-infection occurs to other clients who are on antibiotics.

Precautions should include the use of protective clothing when giving direct care, strict hand hygiene and appropriate cleaning of equipment.

These are just a few examples of infections you are likely to encounter. Your own organization will have developed guidelines on the safe practices which should be taken when caring for clients with infection.

Conclusion

Infection control requires constant vigilance by both individuals and care staff. Much is known about how infections occur and methods of reducing these risks, even of new diseases such as HIV. However, infections continue to remain a problem and claim many lives. The cost is high both in human and monetary terms.

Many infections are preventable both in homes and hospitals, and all individuals carry a responsibility to protect themselves, those with whom they come in contact, and particularly those under their care.

This chapter has stressed the need for the health care worker to adhere to infection control procedures at all times. Health care workers are in a unique position to teach clients and others by their own good example, and to use their knowledge and understanding of infection to play an important role in health education and health promotion.

Points to remember

- Infection is a major problem in all aspects of care.
- The cost to the individual is incalculable in terms of suffering and financial loss.
- Infection costs the taxpayer millions of pounds.
- One out of every three infections is preventable.
- Health and safety of clients is dependent upon application of knowledge in infection control practice.
- Health education and health promotion are paramount in empowering clients.

Practice Activity

Core competence U4 states that you have to contribute to the health, safety and security of individuals and their environment. How can your knowledge of infection control be applied in order to achieve this? Discuss with your supervisor any ideas which you have for improving infection control practice in your own area. If you want further information, try to arrange a meeting with the Infection Control Nurse in your area.

Glossary

Anaphylaxis. An unusual or exaggerated allergic reaction. Substances most likely to produce such reaction include drugs and the venom of bees, wasps and hornets.

CAI. Community-acquired infection.

Colonization. Organisms present and/or multiplying in or on the human body without causing disease.

COSHH. Control of substances hazardous to health.

Disease. "Out of ease".

Endemic. A disease or infection constantly present in the community.

Epidemic. The presence in a population of disease or infection in excess of that usually expected.

HAI. Hospital-acquired infection.

Infection. The entry and multiplication of infectious organisms producing disease in a susceptible person.

Nosocomial infection. Another term for hospital-acquired infection.

Pathogenic. Capable of causing disease.

Pus. A collection of dead tissue, white blood cells and organisms.

Pyrexia. A rise in body temperature above the upper range of normal.

Resident/endogenous organisms. Organisms normally found on the skin and in the body cavities.

Transient organisms. Organisms picked up (mainly on hands) by carers during client care activities and transferred to a susceptible person. Almost all cases of cross-infections can be attributed to transient organisms.

Toxin. A poison.

Further reading

Stucke (1993), Microbiology for Nurses, 7th edn. (Baillière Tindall). This introductory text which is part of the Nurses Aids Series is a comprehensive practical guide to basic microbiology and infection control.

Ayliffe, Collins and Taylor (1990), Hospital Acquired Infection – Principles and Prevention, 2nd edn. (Butterworth–Heinemann). This excellent book touches on most factors associated with some of the common infections encountered in care settings, and care practices which may help prevent or minimize these infections.

Stewart (1993), Skills for Caring (Churchill Livingstone). A small comprehensive book on the importance of hygiene. The range of cover is that of hygiene for both the carer as well as those unable to care for themselves, and environmental hygiene in homes and hospitals. It also includes a section on food handling. A useful companion to other reading material mentioned.

Worsley et al. (eds) (1994), Infection Control – A Community Perspective (Daniels Publishing, Cambridge). Considers the recent changes in the NHS and support service, skillfully moving from hospital-based management to care of the patient in the community.

Campbell (1994), "Making sense of immunity and immunization", Nursing Times, 3 August.

REFERENCES

Ayliffe, G.A.J., Collins, B.J. and Taylor, L.J. (1990). *Hospital Acquired Infection – Principles and Prevention*, 2nd edn (Butterworth–Heinemann).

Currie, E. and Maynard, A. (1989). *Economics of Hospital Acquired Infection*, discussion paper 56, Centre for Health Economics (Health Economics Consortium, University of York, York).

DoH (1992). *Immunization Against Infectious Disease* (HMSO).

Hare, R. and Cooke, E.M. (1984). *Bacteriology and Immunity for Nurses* (Churchill Livingstone).

Ross, K. and Wilson, J.W. (1990). *Anatomy and Physiology in Health and Illness*, 7th edn. (Churchill Livingstone).

HIV and AIDS – attitudes in caring

Peter Wood

Most people have become familiar with the terms HIV and AIDS, through the press, television, posters, leaflets and health education campaigns. However, there is still much confusion and misinformation about HIV and AIDS. In this chapter the terms will be clarified and the difference between them explained.

This chapter explores some of the facts and myths about HIV and AIDS. It looks at these not only in terms of safety and infection control, but also in terms of attitudes to this often misunderstood condition. Although HIV and AIDS are by no means the most important issues in safety and care, they have been the subject of a disproportionate amount of media coverage and discussion. This may mean that either you, your colleagues or your clients are concerned at the dangers presented by HIV and AIDS in the health care setting. For this reason, and to promote greater understanding of these issues, this chapter has been included here.

The key issues of this chapter are:
- The distinction between HIV and AIDS
- Promotion of healthy attitudes towards care of people who are HIV positive
- The role of the health care worker in preventing and controlling the spread of infection.

What is HIV?

HIV stands for **human immunodeficiency virus**, the virus which causes AIDS. HIV is an unusual virus because it attacks and infects the cells of the **immune system**, the body's defence system against disease.

HIV can infect many different cells and tissues, but it seems particularly attracted to the blood cells responsible for coordinating the immune response, the T4 cells. Once inside these cells, HIV may remain dormant for a long time without reproducing. Therefore, a person with HIV may live for many years, possibly 10 or more, without developing symptoms of illness.

This chapter links with Core Unit O, Z8, Y2, U4 and U5.

It is not certain whether everyone with HIV infection will go on to develop related illness.

Most people with HIV will produce **antibodies** to the infection after approximately 3 months; but some will take longer, a year or more, although this is unusual. At this time, they may well have a flu-like illness from which they will soon recover. The antibodies produced seem to be ineffective, leaving HIV free to cause damage to the immune system later.

Eventually HIV becomes reactivated, using the T4 cells almost like factories to produce new viruses. Many T4 cells are damaged in this process and the immune system is weakened, leaving those infected open to many infections, weight loss, night sweats and diarrhoea. This is known as **symptomatic HIV disease**. People with HIV can be seriously ill at this stage, although they will not have an AIDS diagnosis.

What is AIDS?

AIDS stands for **acquired immune deficiency syndrome**. This is the stage of HIV infection where a person's immune system is so badly damaged that it is unable to control many **opportunistic infections** (see Chapter 12). An AIDS diagnosis will only be given when a person develops one or more of the opportunistic infections which has been listed by the Centre of Disease Control in the USA. These include *Pneumocystis carinii* pneumonia, toxoplasmosis, cytomegalovirus and *Mycobacterium* tuberculosis.

Over the past few years, treatments for some of these opportunistic infections have greatly improved, leading to people recovering and having periods of relatively good health in between periods of illness.

Points to remember

- Having HIV is not the same as having AIDS.
- People with HIV may live for many years without developing symptoms of illness.
- You cannot catch AIDS – you can only become infected with HIV.

Promoting healthy attitudes in caring

This section considers the health care worker's role in promoting healthy attitudes to the care of people who have tested HIV-positive, and the factors which may inhibit this process.

Health care workers are well placed to promote healthy attitudes by the example they set. This is demonstrated by the standard of care given.

> **Practice point**
> As a health care worker what does providing a professional service mean to you? Make a list of the factors which you consider to be important.

Some of the things you may have considered are:

- All clients are entitled to the same quality of care.
- Care should be non-judgmental.
- There is an obligation to educate others.

People with HIV have not always been treated in this professional way, and there are two main reasons for this. The first reason is **fear** – fear about HIV and AIDS through lack of knowledge, and fear about sexuality and the culture of intravenous (IV) drug use. These fears are often manifested in judgement. The second reason is that some people consider HIV and AIDS to be **moral issues**.

HIV and AIDS have created much fear generally, and in health care workers much of this is caused by lack of knowledge and understanding, particularly about how HIV is transmitted. Gaining knowledge and understanding are positive ways of overcoming fear.

There are three main ways in which HIV is transmitted. These are:

- by having unprotected (without using a condom) sexual intercourse with an HIV-positive person
- blood-to-blood contact (e.g. through infected hypodermic syringes and needles)
- from HIV-positive mothers to their babies, before birth, during birth or through breast-feeding.

There is no danger of becoming infected with HIV from everyday social contact. Therefore all the following are safe:

- shaking hands and hugging
- kissing
- using toilets
- sharing cups, cutlery and crockery
- sharing bed linen
- sharing food

HIV and AIDS, particularly in the west, have been linked with certain groups, especially gay men and IV drug users. However, in New York City one out of every 64 babies is born HIV-positive; in Los Angeles the ratio is 1:100 and in Edinburgh it is 1:254. *All* sexually active individuals have the potential to be infected and to infect others.

Although sexuality and IV drug-use may be difficult areas for some people to talk about, people's differences should be acknowledged and we should try to understand the complex reasons for people behaving as they do. Acknowledging the diversity of people helps us to see beyond the stereotypes, which are often based on fear. It is often easier to be aware of other people's prejudice than your own.

Points to remember

- You cannot be infected with HIV from everyday social contact.

■ Everyone has a right to care that is non-judgmental, compassionate and of a high quality.

■ It is our fears and attitudes which can get in the way of providing a professional service.

> **Think about**
>
> Attitudes and feelings can often affect the way in which we relate to others. What are your thoughts, feelings and attitudes about each of the following:
>
> ▷ a 25-year-old HIV-positive gay man
> ▷ a 30-year-old female HIV-positive IV drug user
> ▷ a 19-year-old HIV positive haemophiliac
> ▷ a 2-year-old HIV-positive child
> ▷ a 35-year-old HIV-positive mother of three children.
>
> Consider these carefully. What are the similarities and differences? Are there any thoughts, feelings or attitudes identified that could affect the standard of care you would be able to offer each of these people?
>
> It might be helpful to discuss your thoughts and feelings with a friend or colleague.

Preventing and controlling spread

This section considers the role of health care workers in the prevention and control of the spread of infection. There are two main ways in which the health care worker can help. The first of these is through following good infection control procedures, and the second by taking an active role as a health educator.

Infection control practices

It is not possible to tell who does and who does not have HIV infection simply by looking. In some situations you will know that you are working with HIV-positive clients, but in others you won't, as even the clients themselves may be unaware. For this reason it is important to follow universal precautions. As well as protecting you against HIV, they will protect you against hepatitis B and other infections (see also chapter 12).

■ Cuts and abrasions should be covered with a waterproof dressing.

■ Gloves and disposable aprons should always be worn when handling blood or body fluids.

■ Always wash hands thoroughly after removing gloves.

■ Spillage of blood and body fluids should be covered with paper towels and washed with a detergent. Chlorine-releasing granules could be used, or alternatively use a solution of sodium hypochlorite. Always wear gloves when dealing with spillage. If you are working in the community then diluted household bleach is a good alternative.

■ Follow normal procedures for dealing with blood-soaked linen. Linen

contaminated in the community should be washed in the hot cycle of a washing machine (normally 70 degrees or above).
∎ Keep up to date with the infection control policy of your workplace.

Health education role

As yet there is no cure for HIV infection or AIDS. Therefore, education is the only means of prevention available at present. Your work with clients may provide you with opportunities for health education, particularly if they approach you about their concerns or for advice.

These situations should be handled with sensitivity, especially if the discussions are about sexual practice or intravenous drug use. You need to be aware of safer sexual practices and safer drug use.

Points to remember

∎ Always use a condom for penetrative sex.
∎ Encourage exploration of alternatives to penetrative sex.
∎ Never share needles and syringes.
∎ Encourage exploration of alternative drug use.

Your local Health Promotion Service or voluntary agencies working around HIV and drug issues will be able to offer further information and advice.

Think about

Gary is a 31-year-old gay man. He was diagnosed as having AIDS two-and-a-half years ago. Since his first diagnosis of *Pneumocystis carinii* pneumonia (PCP) he has also received treatment for cytomegalovirus (CMV) and toxoplasmosis. He is now extremely weak, has poor mobility and has bouts of prolonged diarrhoea. At present he is being cared for at home, mainly by his partner Jon. On your first two visits to provide care, you notice that Jon does not wear disposable gloves or aprons when dealing with body fluids and that spillages are simply wiped up with a cloth.
▷ How do you feel?
▷ What would you think?
▷ What would you do?
Discuss your responses with a colleague or friend.

There are many possible reasons why Jon does not wear gloves or aprons when dealing with body fluids. He might lack knowledge of correct infection control procedures. He might not have access to disposable gloves and aprons. He might feel that wearing gloves and aprons is inappropriate in the context of his relationship with Gary. Whatever the reason, it is important that the matter be dealt with in a caring and sensitive manner. If you are unsure about how to proceed, seek advice from your supervisor or manager.

Conclusion

The aim of this chapter has been to highlight some important issues which may arise in the care of a person who is HIV-positive. There is no known cure for AIDS, so all health care workers have an important role in helping to prevent the spread of this devastating disease. By setting a good example, and by using knowledge and understanding of infection, the health care worker can assist in the health education of clients and promote safe and healthy lifestyles as well as healthy attitudes.

Finally, as a publication of the American Medical Association put it:

'A person who is afflicted with AIDS needs competent, compassionate treatment. Neither those who have the disease nor those who have been infected with the virus should be subjected to discrimination based on fear or prejudice, least of all by members of the health care community.'

Points to remember

■ Universal precautions protect you from a range of infections as well as HIV.
■ Always use universal precautions even when those around you do not.
■ Sensitivity is needed when dealing with health education in particular around the issues of HIV.

Further reading

Many leaflets have been produced about HIV and AIDS. You will be able to obtain some from your local health education/health promotion service.

Yelding (ed) (1990), Caring for Someone with AIDS. (Consumers Association/Hodder & Stoughton). This is a practical guide for people coping with AIDS. It details where to go for information and support.

Tavanyar (1992), The Terrence Higgens Trust HIV/AIDS Book (Thorsons). Good, clear information about HIV and AIDS, including risk reduction, safer sex, medical, social and political developments; realities of living with HIV and AIDS.

Scott (update twice-yearly), The National AIDS Manual (NAM Publications). This is a comprehensive book in three volumes. Not a book to buy, but good for digging into. It is probably available in your local hospital library or health promotion service library. Volume 1 includes prevention, routes of transmission, safer sex, testing. Volume 2 includes a comprehensive directory of services for people with HIV/AIDS. Volume 3 covers treatments and trials.

Practice activity
Contact your local health Promotion Service or Voluntary HIV and AIDS organization. Find out what resources they have, services offered and any courses they run for health care workers.

SECTION
Rehabilitation and support:
the multidisciplinary team

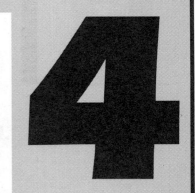

Introduction

Rehabilitation is the process of restoring a person's ability to live and work as normally as possible following a disabling injury or illness. It aims to help the person achieve maximum possible physical and psychological fitness and regain the ability to care for himself or herself.

A team approach is vital in rehabilitation. The "team" is not a fixed entity – its composition varies according to need, but will usually include a doctor, a physiotherapist, occupational therapist and a nurse, as well as support workers. It is the function of the team to improve the mismatch that exists between the client and his or her environment by whatever means necessary.

This section will prove an insight into the roles of the physiotherapist (Chapter 15), occupational therapist (Chapter 14), the nurse and the support worker in relation to rehabilitation. In addition a brief outline of the development of occupational therapy and physiotherapy as professions is given. The inclusion of pain physiology (Chapter 16) is highly relevant to this particular section, and will relate to many other aspects of care.

Finally, Chapter 17 looks at the management of continence. An inability to control bladder and/or bowel function is extremely distressing for any individual. The support worker, through knowledge, understanding and patience, can help the individual to regain continence – which in turn will have a positive effect on their psychological and physical fitness.

14 | Occupational therapy

Joanna Fogden and Anita Wood

Occupational therapists and their support workers are important members of the multidisciplinary team, using occupation or purposeful activity to promote rehabilitation.

The idea of using purposeful activity to promote rehabilitation is not new, and has been used by doctors since before 600 BC to improve the well-being of both the body and the mind. This emphasis on mental and physical interdependence is one of the fundamental principles of occupational therapy today.

The professional status of occupational therapy developed during and after the Second World War when many young men returned from the fighting suffering from physical injuries and psychological trauma. These men needed rehabilitation and help in returning to a useful and productive life. The popular belief was that basket weaving was the main activity taught by occupational therapists at this time, but in fact their involvement in the rehabilitation process was extensive. Today the occupational therapist works in a wide range of health care, including physical rehabilitation, mental health, paediatrics, learning difficulties, in community settings, in prisons, with young offenders, hospices and many others.

For the purposes of this book some specific activities, where the support worker is involved, have been chosen.

The key issues of this chapter are:
- Client assessment
- Activities of living
- Practising how to dress
- The home visit

This chapter links with the O unit and endorsements X14, X15.

Client assessment

Assessment of the client is the most important skill of the occupational therapist but every member of the multidisciplinary team can contribute to the assessment.

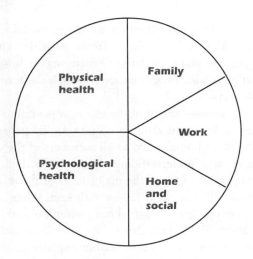

Figure 14.1   Assessing the whole person

The assessment is of *the whole person*, and as in all other aspects of care must take into account the client's physical, psychological and psychosocial well-being (see Figure 14.1). The team approach to assessment is important in ensuring that the client will achieve maximum independence.

You will meet clients who are away from their normal environment, but the whole team will be working to allay their anxieties and help them to achieve their goals.

There may be a number of reasons why a person is unable to cope with self-care. Reasons include a prolonged stay in hospital due to a medical or surgical problem, an acute confusional state, multiple social problems, or disability.

Rehabilitation usually starts in hospital where the client's immediate health problems are stabilized and an assessment is made prior to planning a rehabilitation programme. The client may remain in an acute area of the hospital, but ideally should be moved so that the benefits of the consistent policy of a rehabilitation ward may be made available.

It is not always possible for a person undergoing rehabilitation to return to the community and independent living. During the rehabilitation process, assessments are made to establish how much support a person may require in the future – and for some this will mean being cared for in a residential or nursing home. People with chronic disease are largely cared for at home where the community physiotherapist, community occupational therapist and the district nurse will be involved with rehabilitation.

For the client admitted to a hospital rehabilitation unit or ward, their individuality is of prime importance. No two individuals will have the same requirements for everyday living, and their expectations will not be the same. For that reaason activities should be structured to individual requirements but flexible enough to allow for unexpected change. The client's needs will change continually, so regular reassessments should be made and care adjusted accordingly.

The client admitted to a rehabilitation ward has usually had any medical condition investigated and made stable as far as possible. There may still be multiple problems but the main reason for remaining in hospital is to regain lost skills. Rehabilitation is a learning situation in which the learning is broken up into small achievable steps.

To be able to make an assessment of the client, it is vital to get to know him or her as well as possible. Good communication skills are essential. No one person is with the client 24 hours a day, so all members of the care team should share their knowledge and understanding of the individual, to build up as complete a picture as possible. One of the major roles of the nurse is in ensuring that everyone involved with the client liaises with each other.

The assessment itself is usually carried out through observing and questioning the client in a variety of different situations. The client must be included in this process and the reasons for this observation explained. The client's wishes and ideas must be respected, and relatives or carers should also be asked for their views or ideas.

Following a general assessment, a **rehabilitation programme** is planned for the individual, aiming for a balance between all sides of the client's life – that is, home, work, family and leisure; to preserve function by the provision of aids and adaptations; and to prevent unnecessary deterioration by educating the client in the most sensible management of problems.

A more specific assessment looks at the **activities of daily living**.

Areas of assessment

The following headings are broad and in some cases will need to be more specific to the individual client.

- *Personal care*: washing; using the toilet; eating; dressing.
- *Mobility*: walking; transferring (from chair to bed); need for a wheelchair?
- *Dexterity*: reaching; lifting; carrying; handling.
- *Home conditions*: type of house (flat, bungalow, house, ?stairs); housework; shopping; cooking; cleaning.
- *Work*.
- *Social and leisure activities*.
- *Communication*: eyesight; hearing; writing ability; understanding; speech.
- *Personality and mental state*: anxious or relaxed; dependent or independent; positive or negative attitude?

Although such a detailed assessment will be carried out by a qualified member of the OT team, the support worker will be able to provide additional information through working closely with the client. True feelings and reactions are often revealed when not under direct observation.

In hospital, client assessment will give consideration to the following.

Think about

Think about all the activities you do in a day from getting up in the morning to going to bed at night. Your "list" of activities may be quite long, but you will probably have taken the ability to do basic things for granted.

Ability to maintain a safe environment

If the client is initially unable to move, particular care is needed in positioning and handling. Nurses and support workers undergo instruction in lifting and handling techniques and in the use of wheelchairs, to ensure maximum safety for the client and the carer. The client must be protected from falling or injury.

Chairs and tables should be at the correct height, personal requirements within easy reach, and most importantly an effective system of summoning help must be at hand. A disabled person is restricted and may not fully realize his or her limitations.

Communication

In our everyday lives, communication is through speech, hearing, vision and non-verbal signs. If one sense is reduced the sensitivity of the remaining senses is heightened, and the client may have to learn to communicate in new ways. The client may be unable to speak but understands; may have limited vocabulary; or may be unable to understand anything. In each case a method of communicating should be initiated at the first meeting with the client. Gestures and non-verbal communication are often very effective, but if the client does not speak English a translator is essential.

The client may be referred to the speech and language therapist, who will be able to judge whether he/she would benefit from speech therapy.

Establishing effective communication enables the nurse and support worker to better understand the client's comprehension of his or her condition, and enables the client to express needs and wishes. Extra time is needed to communicate. The willingness of staff to sit and listen to the client's worries, to accept and understand without censure, will go a long way in helping to reduce anxiety.

Ability to eat and drink

Mealtimes have an important social and psychological significance in everyone's day. For clients with a disability the apparently simple task of eating may pose numerous problems.

All clients should be encouraged and helped in choosing their menu. This often provides the opportunity to give information about diet, and advice on eating a healthy diet at home. Always maintain the client's dignity by ensuring that clothes are protected from spillage and that sufficient time is given to eat, and encourage the client to feed himself or herself as much as possible. The occupational therapist can provide advice on **aids and adaptations** which may make eating and drinking easier.

For some clients swallowing is difficult, and this may make them reluctant to eat. Advice from the dietitian can be sought regarding foods that are both palatable and easily swallowed. Gradually over time independence will increase.

Elimination

Loss of independent control of bladder and/or bowel often causes a great deal of anxiety and depression in clients. Many older clients may believe that such

> **Practice point**
> The next time you sit down to eat a meal, use only one hand. You may find this quite easy, but give some thought to levels of difficulty depending on what food is on the plate. How do you think you might feel if someone fed you? Ask a friend or colleague to sit with you at a meal and feed you. Now how do you feel?

Think about
How would you feel if
you had to wear
nightclothes all day?
You would probably feel
rather depersonalized
and conspicuous.

problems are due to their age and that nothing can be done. Chapter 17 gives further information on how to help people regain continence.

Information from the client about their normal patterns of elimination will be needed, as prolonged periods of immobility and disability will interfere with normal function. Clients may be quite embarrassed to talk about this subject, so any discussion should be sensitive and private.

Personal cleaning and dressing

Clients usually feel better when they are dressed in their normal clothing. Clothes should be simple, light and loose, but as far as possible clients should wear what they find most comfortable. A well-fitting pair of shoes is more comfortable and safer then floppy slippers. Encourage clients to choose for themselves what they would like to wear, ensuring that the clothes are clean.

Washing and dressing may be carried out at the bedside, or in the bathroom area; *but wherever this activity takes place dignity and privacy must be respected*. Men should not be left unshaven, and women should be allowed to wear makeup if they choose. More information on dressing practice is given later in this chapter.

Mobility and independence

Limitation of **mobility** may be due to a number of different problems. In some conditions, pain may be the limiting factor, in others muscle weakness. Each client will have a different combination of deficits, so the techniques involved in helping to improve mobility will vary with each client.

The basis for treatment is always set on a thorough understanding of *normal movement patterns*. Therefore it is worth while establishing from the client how mobile and active they were prior to their disability or illness. This information helps in the setting of **realistic and achievable goals** – otherwise you might inadvertently expect the client to be participating in the next London marathon!

Regular and frequent discussions with other members of the team are needed, *to ensure that everyone is giving the client consistent information*. If a client is assisted to walk in a manner different from that taught by the physiotherapist he will become confused and possibly unstable. This puts the client and others at risk. Nurses, support workers, physiotherapists, occupational therapists and the client must work in harmony, gradually encouraging a greater degree of independence.

Work and leisure

For many people a disabling illness will mean a loss of employment and possibly financial hardship. This in itself can exacerbate frustration and social isolation, and lead to additional strain on self-esteem. The client and their family may need very specific advice and help from the social worker. Worries over work and finance should never be underestimated.

For clients who have a prolonged stay in hospital the days can become monotonous and boring. On finding out what interests and hobbies they have, efforts can be made to continue these. Obviously some hobbies such as DIY or fly-fishing are unsuitable for a hospital environment; but with a little bit of careful thought and ingenuity a variety of suitable activities can be arranged. The support worker should spend time with the client – listening, supporting, encouraging new skills and perhaps playing games which are therapy in disguise.

People vary in how much they value **social contact**; but for those for whom it is important, visits and participation by a supportive network of family and close friends is to be encouraged. Relatives may be invited to attend treatment sessions to see for themselves how progress is made and to give them the opportunity to learn how to care for the client on their return home. Social interchange between the clients on the ward is also important, and people with similar problems often provide support for each other. The families, too, can forge friendships, gaining strength and comfort during a difficult time.

Hospital wards tend to be busy bustling places, but every effort should be made to allow clients and their visitors some **privacy**. Young people are perhaps less inhibited than elderly people about hugging their partner in public, so staff should be sensitive to a client's need. Physical contact with a loved one is often very reassuring and comforting.

Sleep and rest

Sleep patterns inevitably alter in hospital. A strange bed, unfamiliar surroundings and noise will all affect the ability to sleep, but a restful sleep at night will enable the client to cope with the daily activities. Each of us has our own particular routine, and clients should go to bed and rise in the morning at the times they would normally at home. People who are night workers may find it difficult to adjust to being awake during the day. Ensuring that the client is pain-free, comfortable and as relaxed as possible will all aid restful sleep. For clients who are immobile, helping them to change position regularly will relieve pressure areas and make them more comfortable. Some people may like to catnap during the day, and often feel refreshed after a short snooze. Where possible activities should be worked around the client's routine.

The overall picture

All the issues discussed above are interlinked, and although they are by no means comprehensive they are areas on which the support worker has an impact. To a large extent rehabilitation is "hands off ". It is important to observe what the client *can* do and to stand back, intervening only when really necessary. For many carers this is difficult. Relate this to the "nurturing parent ego-state" in Chapter 4 which, when overused, may take over and disallow the individual from developing skills. Allow clients to go at their own pace even with the simplest of tasks, and they and the team will be rewarded with a sense of achievement.

Families and people who are significant to the client are also considered to be part of the care team. At first they may be distraught about their relative and have difficulty in understanding how the illness or disability will affect the family unit in the future. It is important to have some indication of the family's characters, strengths, weaknesses and roles, and to find out about the client's and the family's expectations. A sound, trusting relationship needs to be established between the carers. The family may need emotional recharging, practical help and guidance in sorting out problems and support. The giving of information about progress is important – provided there is no conflict with confidentiality – as it often helps relieve some anxieties.

Hospital can become an extension of the home. Pleasant, quiet surroundings, with happy, smiling, courteous people, will act as an encouragement to the client to achieve goals.

As a client's condition improves, opportunities will be taken to start integrating him or her into the community. Visits outside the hospital will be arranged. This may involve a visit home for a few hours or overnight. Planning for a client's discharge is not arranged immediately before discharge, it is initiated on admission to hospital. This allows for planning and discussion between the hospital and community care teams to ensure that, on discharge, all the required services will be in place. This is not always easy, but it highlights the need for all team members to communicate with each other. The social worker may be involved in arranging financial assistance, grants for house alterations, day care or home care. The district nurse may need to visit regularly, and volunteer services may be called upon to provide additional support such as visiting schemes or transport.

Not all clients spend prolonged periods in hospital. Some people who suffer from a chronic disabling condition may spend very short spells in hospital or be cared for through the hospital's outpatient department, where the multidisciplinary team continues to help the client maintain functional ability and independence.

Occupational therapy in rehabilitation

> **Think about**
>
> Imagine that you are a 55-year-old woman with longstanding rheumatoid arthritis. Your eyesight is poor and you have difficulty in lifting your arms to put in your eyedrops.
>
> You have recently been widowed. Your husband used to help with the shopping, housework and cooking. Now you live alone in a three-bedroom house with a large garden. Your family are grown up and live some distance away. However, you are anxious to be as independent as possible and would like to develop some hobbies and leisure interests.
>
> ▷ What would *your* priorities be?
> ▷ Which problem would you most want solving?
> ▷ Ask a friend or colleague the same question. Are your answers the same?

Different people react in different ways to the same situation. One person may be happy to move to a small bungalow or ground-floor flat, but another may be reluctant to leave the home in which they have spent all their married life and raised their children. We must never make assumptions about what a person wishes, so we must establish what the client wishes to do and help to solve major difficulties. The final plan is a collaboration between the client and the therapist and should be agreeable to both sides.

On completion of the assessment, an individual programme is planned. It may include:

- dressing practice
- training therapy to encourage the client to reach maximum functional ability
- a home assessment visit
- psychological support for the client, their family and carers
- leisure activities.

Dressing practice

Dressing practice – as opposed to "getting the client dressed" – is part of the treatment programme and will be directed by the occupational therapist.

One of the aims of the therapy programme is the transition from *dependence* to *independence*. This is particularly important if the client lives alone, and it also relieves the burden upon carers. All members of the team must recognize this and encourage the client to use the planned techniques at all times. Try not to give any more help than is absolutely necessary.

Some of the techniques referred to in this section relate particularly to people who have had a stroke, for they require the most complete rehabilitation. Many individual techniques will, however, be appropriate in other situations such as with rheumatoid arthritis, elderly care, and orthopaedics (joint replacement/ amputation).

Dressing is a well-learned task and has the advantage of being both practical and visual. It also gives the client a great sense of self-esteem as goals are achieved.

When should dressing practice begin?

It should begin as soon as the client is able to sit out of bed for a reasonable time. For a client who has had a stroke, there should be head control, some degree of trunk control and therefore adequate sitting balance. Practice should take place at the appropriate time of day.

For some client groups (e.g. rheumatoid arthritis) difficulties will probably be limited to one or two problem areas which can be tackled at any time appropriate to the individual. For example, a client having treatment in the hydrotherapy pool will need a change of clothing, and this opportunity can be used.

Where should dressing take place?

It should be done in the normal place, beside the bed or in the bathroom. Privacy and dignity for the client are paramount. One client remarked that following a lengthy stay in hospital he "would cheerfully sit on a commode outside the high street shops without turning a hair!" Curtains and screens should be drawn, doors closed and all personal and private activities should remain personal and private.

Basic principles of dressing

The client should sit on a chair of suitable height with hips and knees at 90 degrees (right angle). This reduces spasm or tension in the limbs. If balance is a problem the client may feel more secure with another chair placed alongside, or sitting on the bed.

The affected limb is placed into a garment first when dressing, and comes out last when undressing. This is because it is easier, as there is more material to work with. The limb may be affected by a stroke, arthritis, injury or recent surgery. In general the clothing should be loose rather than tight-fitting.

In the early stages dress the top half first, then the lower half – as this means standing only once. With good functional return the client can then be encouraged to adopt a more normal dressing routine.

Positioning of affected limb(s) must be considered, to promote symmetry, correct limb positioning, and to avoid abnormal patterns of movement relating to the affected side.

The participation of the client is continuously upgraded from passive to active involvement, with assistance decreasing in line with recovery. It is inevitable that there will be times when the client becomes frustrated, tired and demotivated. Providing verbal prompts, visual demonstration, lots of encouragement and praise will help. Do not make the client feel rushed, allow plenty of time at first and reduce it as the client becomes more able to cope.

For activities such as brushing the teeth and combing the hair, the client can be provided with small adaptations which will help. Extended handles are useful for hairbrushes or toothbrushes, particularly for people who cannot raise their arm very high. For cleaning false teeth the client can use a suction brush. An electric razor for shaving is easier than trying to wet-shave. For women who would normally use makeup, choose cosmetics which are easy to apply.

The client should, at each stage, be left looking as good as possible, but be alert to the possibility that a client who has suffered a stroke may be quite shocked to view their appearance in a mirror.

Early independence should not be achieved "at all costs". Too many new methods to learn at once will simply confuse and discourage the client when they fail or forget. Think back to Chapter 8 on Learning Disabilities – on the need to set achievable goals and to take things one step at a time. The same rules apply here. It is best to take things slowly and to concentrate on the problems which the client feels are most important.

The home visit

When a hospital patient has recovered sufficient functional independence, and discharge is being considered, a home visit may be planned to assess the client's abilities in their own setting. This permits an appraisal of the layout and facilities in the home.

Think about

Imagine that you have a broken arm – you can make it even more difficult if you imagine that it is your dominant arm. What do you think your difficulties would be? Think back to the earlier question about all the activities you do in a day.

Now try to put on a jumper. Can you work out the best way of coping? Don't cheat!

When you have mastered that, imagine that you have both your arm and your leg incapacitated and put on a pair of tights or trousers. How frustrated did this make you feel? Did you identify any other emotions?

You will probably experience a range of emotions – anger, frustration and irritation to name but a few – and it is important for you to acknowledge similar emotions in your clients.

Practice point

Should an opportunity arise for you to spend some time with an occupational therapist, then do so, and ask to observe a dressing assessment or practice session. Make sure you also ask the client if you might observe.

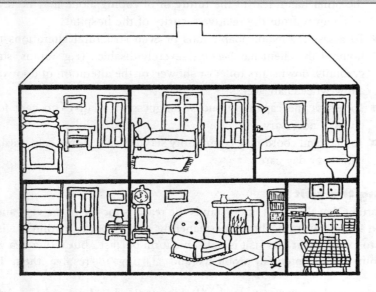

Figure 14.2   Appraising the layout and facilities in the home

Usually two members of staff accompany the client on the home visit, both for the safety of the client and as legal protection for the staff in the event of any complaint – a situation which is extremely rare.

The occupational therapist acts as the key team member. The accompanying staff member may be the physiotherapist, if mobility is a problem, a social worker if there are social problems, or a nurse or support worker if home nursing may be required. The members of staff involved are those whose experience is most suited to the needs of the client.

Members of other caring organizations may also be involved (e.g. the home care organizer). Where major adaptations are needed the community occupational therapist should be invited to attend the home visit.

The aims of the home visit

- To ease the transfer from hospital to community life.
- To gain an insight into the circumstances a client will have to cope with following discharge.
- To provide the therapist with the opportunity to assess how the client will cope alone or with the help of relatives.
- To ensure that the aids and adaptations planned in hospital can be used equally well at home (a walking frame may be easy to manoeuvre in an open ward but not so easy to manage in a cluttered cottage with narrow passages).
- To be sensitive to the client's emotional reactions to the possibility of discharge. Once surrounded by familiar objects the client may be more prepared to cope than in the unfamiliar surroundings of a hospital. On the other hand, fear of the future or of coping alone may be revealed when away from the relative security of the hospital.
- To assess for major adaptations or even structural alterations to the home if the client has become severely disabled (e.g. ramps, stairlift, grabrails, downstairs toilet or shower, or the alteration of doorways to allow wheelchair access).
- To assess the capability and willingness of relatives to care for the client if necessary.
- To plan and coordinate community services (e.g. home help, meals-on-wheels or day care).

Planning the visit

It is important that the client understands the reasons for the home visit and that he or she is not returning home permanently at this point in time. It is also essential to explain that this visit is not some form of "test", but rather is a way of finding out about potential problems and starting to resolve them before discharge.

Relatives and carers must also be closely involved and permission obtained to visit the house.

A basic "Home Visit Kit" will include:

- the address, clear directions, road map and most importantly a key for the house
- loose change for the telephone
- the hospital phone number
- a notebook and tape measure
- tea, coffee, milk etc. for a kitchen assessment
- a self-discharge form just in case the client refuses to return to the hospital
- polythene bags and tissues in case of travel sickness
- any necessary equipment (e.g. raised toilet seat, grab rails or bath aids).

Ensure that the client has suitable outdoor clothing and shoes, and if possible arrange to meet representatives of community services during the visit, as this saves time on phone calls later.

During the visit

Although each visit has its own special problems, there are some general points to look for.

Access

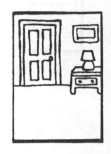

Gate – can the client open it?
Path – is it sloping, is the surface even?
Steps – how many; are they steep?
Door key – can the client open the door?
Lifts – can the client operate the lift?

The Hall

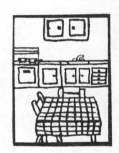

Is there enough room to manoeuvre?
Can the client walk round with a frame, or self-propel the wheelchair?
Rugs – should they be removed?
Light switches/sockets – are they accessible?
Thresholds – are they secure?
Telephone – is it in a convenient place; can the client sit down to use it?

The Living Room

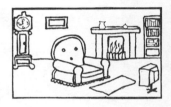

Are the seats easy to get in and out of?
Is the carpet worn; are rugs a potential hazard?
Furniture – is there space to move easily around; does it offer some support?
Appliances – radio, TV, fire: can they be switched on and off with ease?

The Kitchen

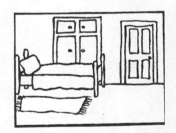

Cupboards – can their contents be reached?
Sink/taps – is the sink a suitable height; can the taps be turned?
Kettle/fridge/cooker – can they be used safely?
Work surfaces – are they the right height?
Are any aids needed?

The Bedroom

The bed – is it the correct height; are the bed covers manageable?
Is there enough space to move round the room?
Can the client manage the lights/heating?

The Bathroom

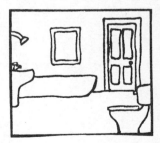

Can the client get in and out of the bath independently; would a shower be better?
Will a raised toilet seat be needed, or would a commode be more suitable?
Where is the best place to site grab rails?

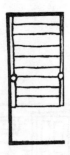

The Stairs

Up/down – is assistance required?

Carpet – is it loose or worn?

Lighting – is there sufficient light?

Bannisters/rails – are they secure and at the correct height?

After the visit

The occupational therapist will compile a full report setting out the present situation, level of independence, actions to be taken and any concerns regarding potential risks. The report is filed in the client's notes and copies are forwarded to all parties involved – this may include the GP, relatives and in many cases the client too.

The home visit may be a very straightforward affair, such as ensuring that the client will be safe and fitting some simple adaptations. Or the visit may highlight major problems and lead to a very specific programme of rehabilitation.

Example

Ann suffered a stroke which left her blind and partially para-lysed, and she was diabetic. You might believe that with so

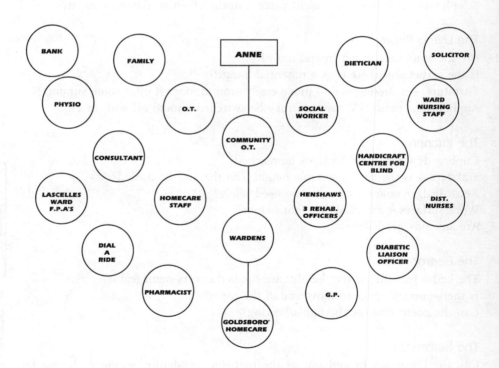

Figure 14.3 Anne's support network

many health problems it would be impossible for her to live independently in the community.

As Anne had spent several years in a Young Disabled Unit her ambition was to live in a place of her own, and when suitable accommodation was found her rehabilitation programme was adapted to meet her future needs. Regular practice in a full-size kitchen within the occupational therapy department, interspersed with visits to the flat, were highlights of Anne's week. She learned to cope with the door intercom, use the telephone and prepare simple meals in her own kitchen. Trips to the supermarket were exciting and Anne was encouraged to take an active part in selecting and buying food. Eventually, with the help of a great many people, health care specialists and others (see Figure 14.3), Anne moved into her own flat where she lived happily and successfully.

John, on the other hand, was quite independent around the house, but there was one snag: his arthritis made it difficult to open his front door. A simple adaptation attached to the door key solved the problem and he was once again self-reliant.

Thus, it can be as complex as a whole lifestyle or as simple as a door key.

Points to remember

- Whatever type of disability a person may suffer, normal everyday life will change.
- Individuals will respond in different ways, but the response may be similar to that of mourning, where the client progresses through reactions of depression, anger, irritability and rejection.
- In some instances, independent living will be difficult or impossible, giving rise to lowered self-esteem and vulnerability.
- Not all problems and difficulties can be dealt with, but adequate assessment of the disabilities arising from illness or injury, by the team, will lead to improved management and go a long way to solving the problems.

Practice Activity

You may be able to accompany an occupational therapist on a home visit. Before the visit talk to the client and sensitively find out as much as you can about their home circumstances. Think about possible problems from this information.

After the visit, assess the accuracy of your predictions. How realistic was the client? Were there any surprises or unforeseen problems?

Further reading

Jay (1985), Help Yourselves (Butterworth). A handbook for hemiplegics and their families. Although written specifically for people who have had a stroke, many of the techniques apply to a wider range of disabilities. A user-friendly reference book.

Eggers (1991), Occupational Therapy in the treatment of the Adult Hemiplegic (Heinemann). Has some excellent ideas on suitable individual and group activities.

Irvine, Bagnall, Smith and Bishop (1993), The Older Patient – An introduction to Geriatric Nursing (Hodder & Stoughton). Primarily a nursing textbook, it also has good line drawings of aids and adaptations, especially in the chapters on dressing, eating and personal care. Chapters on the principles and techniques of rehabilitation emphasize the multidisciplinary approach.

The Disabled Living Foundation (380–384 Harrow Road, London W9 2HV) publishes notes on all aspects of daily living – for example, Dressing for Disabled People by Rosemary Ruston.

The role of the physiotherapist | 15

Fiona Evard

The physiotherapist, working with other members of the care team, is involved in helping individuals to achieve maximum physical and psychological fitness following injury, surgery, medical or mental illness.

The first chapter of this section has looked at the aims of rehabilitation and the roles of the nurse, the occupational therapist and the support worker as members of the multidisciplinary team.

The key issues for this chapter are:
- The role of the physiotherapist
- Methods of treatment
- Assessment
- The role of the support worker or physiotherapy helper

Origins of the profession

The practice of "physical therapy" was initiated by two nurses, Rosalind Paget and Lucy Robinson, who set up the Society of Trained Masseuses in 1894. "Medical rubbing", as it was then known, was gradually recognized as a legitimate treatment. From simple massage, a variety of treatment techniques were developed over the years, including remedial exercises, medical gymnastics and medical electricity.

Many of the advances that have been made within rehabilitation practice have evolved from the knowledge and experience of treating people injured in wars.

Along with advances in treatments, the training and education of physiotherapists has become more widespread. Today there are more than 25 000 physiotherapists registered with the Society of Chartered Physiotherapists. Physiotherapy is just one of the specialties allied to medicine, and as such will be found in a variety of settings both inside and outside the hospital (see Figure 15.1).

This chapter links with the O Unit, U4, U3 and endorsement units X10, X11, X13, Z7, X8, X9, X10.

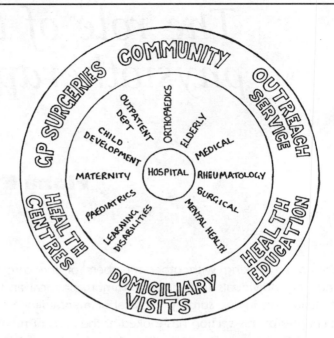

Figure 15.1 The specialties applied to rehabilitation

The role of the physiotherapist

The definition of physiotherapy from the Chartered Society is:

> A systematic method of assessing musculoskeletal and neurological disorders of function, including pain and those of psychological origin, and treating or preventing these problems by natural methods based essentially on manual practice and physical agencies.

The physical means will be examined first. Many of the treatments described are carried out by the physiotherapist in a hospital outpatient department. For those who are unable to travel, the physiotherapist will go into the community to provide domiciliary care.

Everyone is familiar with the sight of physiotherapists on the football pitch, helping injured players. Perhaps it is not so well known that they also work with brain-damaged children, encouraging them to develop as normally as possible. The support provided for children and their parents is invaluable and will often continue for many years as these children grow to become adolescents.

Amputees undergo a tremendous amount of rehabilitation before and after surgery. It is important that as soon as their stump has healed they mobilize well. Even before their own artificial limb has been measured and made, a temporary limb can be fitted and walking can begin under careful supervision.

Perhaps you have had physiotherapy following a sports injury or a fracture. Perhaps an elderly relative has had heat treatment for painful joints or exercise following a stroke. Wherever there is a client with a physical problem which stops them from leading the sort of life they would wish, the physiotherapist is part of the team that can help.

Exercises

For each client a specific exercise programme is devised and altered according to the client's progress and changing needs. Exercises are used for a variety of reasons:

- to increase muscle power and endurance
- to improve the range of movement in a joint
- to improve neuromuscular coordination
- to improve cardiovascular efficiency
- to re-educate functional activity.

To a large extent, progress is dependent on the efforts of the client, not only when working with the physiotherapist but also when doing the exercises at home.

In many clinics and hospitals the physiotherapist will hold a group exercise class. The clients usually have some common disability or condition which will benefit from similar exercises or activities – for example osteoarthritis or a stiff back. Antenatal and postnatal classes are a well-known example of exercise classes for a specific group of clients.

For most clients, working in a group with other people who have similar problems provides support and encouragement. This is very important in helping the client to overcome fear and sometimes discomfort. Clients need constant,

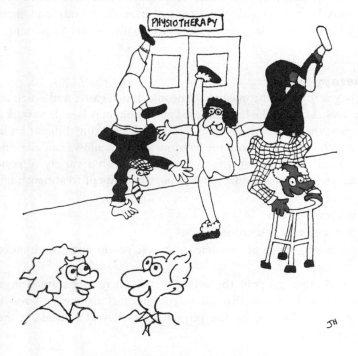

WE FIND THE GROUP EXERCISE CLASS TO BE VERY POPULAR. AS FOR YOUR MOTHER, MR LEE, WELL SHE'S COMING ON IN LEAPS AND BOUNDS.

Practice point
Find out what classes are organized by your local hospital or clinic. If possible ask the physiotherapist if you can join a class. You might be surprised at your own level of fitness.

gentle reminders of their exercises and the support worker plays a vital role in coaxing and encouraging.

Some forms of exercise are termed **passive**. The client's joints are put through a range of movement by the physiotherapist, as opposed to the client controlling movement. A client who is paralysed, for example, will need assistance in moving their arm or leg. Regular passive exercise may help to prevent the joints in a paralysed limb becoming stiff. Should some nerve activity return, it also helps the muscles to work in a normal way and not be too tight or too floppy. The physiotherapist will direct nursing staff, support workers and carers in carrying out passive exercises on particular clients.

Clients suffering from a mental illness are frequently introverted and reluctant to move. Appropriate exercise often enables them to express their feelings and anxieties.

Relaxation

Just as exercise is vital to maintain our musculoskeletal system, relaxation is equally important. People who have difficulty in relaxing often complain of muscle aches and headaches, and generally sleep badly.

There are numerous methods of relaxation. Some use techniques where, by tightening and then relaxing muscles in sequence, it is possible to appreciate the difference and therefore achieve a heightened state of relaxation. Muscles will relax more readily following exercise.

Other techniques of relaxation involve imagining favourite scenes or places, listening to a calming piece of music or poem. Whatever method is chosen, relaxation aims to give an individual control over their body and their mind. Exercise and relaxation, in groups or individually, is an important part of treatment.

Hydrotherapy

Exercising in water is, for the majority of people, much easier and much more fun than on dry land. A client who has restricted movement may be able to walk in water as it counteracts the gravitational forces which make walking difficult on land.

The warmth of the water and the freedom which it allows can give enormous psychological and physical benefits to individuals with a variety of conditions, such as rheumatic or orthopaedic conditions. The aims of treatment include:

- decreasing pain
- promotion of relaxation
- increasing range of movement, muscle power and coordination.

In the hydrotherapy pool the safety of the client is paramount, and the support worker will ensure that all safety precautions are adhered to. The support worker, as directed by the physiotherapist, will also assist the client with their exercises.

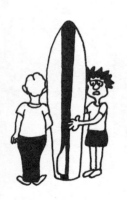

EXCUSE ME, IS THIS THE WAY TO THE HYDROTHERAPY DEPARTMENT?

Think about
Think about the clients you work with. How much exercise do they get? How might safe and appropriate exercise classes be introduced?

Breathing exercises

The definition of physiotherapy mentioned earlier implied that the physiotherapist treats only musculoskeletal or neurological disorders.

However, the physiotherapist is frequently asked to treat disorders of the chest and is regularly seen working with clients who have suffered trauma or surgery. In the intensive care unit the physiotherapist pays meticulous attention to the lungs, making sure that the client's airway remains clear, helping the client to cough, or using mechanical suction to remove secretions if the client is on a ventilator.

For children who have cystic fibrosis, keeping their lungs free of secretions is essential to their survival. The physiotherapist will be closely involved with carers, teaching and supporting them with the exercises and procedures needed to be carried out several times each day.

Manipulation and mobilization

Manipulation and mobilization are frequently used in the treatment of musculoskeletal disorders. Probably the most common condition treated in this way is a back problem. Nurses and support workers in particular, by the very nature of their occupation, are susceptible to problems of the spine and comprise a small proportion of the clients treated by the physiotherapist. To a large extent back problems are preventable.

> ### Point to remember
> Everyone, including nurses and support workers, must ensure that they adhere at all times to the correct procedures for lifting and handling as laid down by the health and safety at work policy.

Massage

Massage as a form of treatment is not used as frequently today as it was in the past. However, it may be used as a means of alleviating oedema in a limb, the limb being elevated during the massage to help drain the excess fluid. In certain localized areas of the body, friction massage may be used to relieve pain, or following skin grafting to increase the circulation to the new skin.

Although massage is often an instinctive way of relieving discomfort, you must be careful about when and how you use it on a client. The physiotherapist will advise you if massage is considered to be a suitable therapeutic treatment.

Massage is used in conjunction with aromatherapy oils and has been shown to be very effective in reducing stress. In health care settings these oils should only be used by someone who has had a recognized training in their use.

Hot and cold therapy

Electrotherapy uses electricity to create heat. The application of heat can be very therapeutic, in that it can stimulate the circulation, relieve pain and relax muscles.

There are various other ways in which heat can be applied. For example, superficial heat can be produced using special packs which are steeped in hot water, then wrapped in towels before being applied to the affected area.

Conducted heat can be applied to the hands and feet by dipping them into hot wax, which is then covered and left to cool.

Electrical current can provide deep heat to the tissues of the body. Specialized equipment is necessary to be able to produce the right amount of heat in exactly the right place, and this form of treatment requires a great deal of skill by the professional.

Just as heat is beneficial, cold therapy also has a place in treatment. Cold therapy is used to relieve pain, reduce oedema and to help muscle activity. The majority of people will have used a "cold compress" at some time, either for the relief of pain or as treatment for a recent sprain to an ankle or wrist.

Other therapies

Other forms of treatment include the use of ultrasound, high-frequency energy, infrared radiation, interferential and combined therapy, which influences the pain-conducting nerve endings, as well as laser therapy and electrical acupuncture.

The assessment

Thorough assessment of the client is vital. It must always be remembered that assessment should take into account not only the physical factors, but also the social, psychological and environmental factors which have an impact on the client. The initial assessment sets the foundation upon which treatment can be designed and progress measured. The physiotherapist will then evaluate the effectiveness of the programme, revising it as necessary.

In many departments the "soap" system is used to record relevant information:

     s = subjective factors
     o = objective factors
     a = aims
     p = plan.

We call these **problem-orientated medical records**.

Subjective factors

What does the *client* think is the problem?
Where does it hurt and when?
Does it interrupt their sleep?
Did any specific incident bring it on?
How long has it been hurting?
What makes it worse?
What makes it better?

Objective factors

What is the diagnosis; i.e. what does the doctor say is wrong?
The first time you are able to observe the client note how he or she moves. The

facial expression will often tell you a lot about the condition in terms of how it is affecting the client.

If X-ray examinations have been done, what do they show?

If there is a painful area, how does it respond to examination?

Is it bruised, tender to the touch, or swollen?

Does what the client tell you match with what you observe?

Aims

What does the client expect from treatment?

What does the physiotherapist expect to gain from the treatment?

Are the expectations realistic?

Decide on common goals and the time scale in which you expect to achieve them.

Plan

How will these goals be achieved?

Which treatment techniques will be used?

How often will the patient need to attend for treatment?

Will they have a regime of home exercises to do?

Does any other health professional need to become involved?

Is a home visit necessary?

Does their partner/parent/relative need information?

Do they have a subsequent appointment to see the Doctor?

Assessment example

Name: John Cooper   *Age*: 28   *M. status*: Married

History of present condition: Eight weeks post-operation, fixing of fracture to right lower leg, sustained whilst playing football. Plaster removed today (18 June 1994) – X-ray shows good position and healing.

Subjective: Mr Cooper is very anxious. Pain-free whilst in plaster but now finds knee and ankle painful. Calf muscle thin. Obtains comfort with foot resting on a stool.

Objective: Well-healed fracture, wasted calf muscle, walking poor with two sticks. Deep bruising evident around the ankle. *Movements*: ankle flexion = 15°, extension = 10°, inversion = 5°, eversion = 0°; knee full range; weak thigh muscles.

On palpation: ankle thick and some degree of swelling present. Pain score = 5/10. Client is reluctant to bear weight on heel and limps markedly. Although anxious he is well-motivated and will do well.

Client's aims:

■ Play football a.s.a.p.

■ Drive car

■ Go walking in Tibet in 3 months' time.

Physiotherapy aims:
(1) Reduce pain around fracture site.
(2) Restore mobility to ankle joint.
(3) Increase muscle power in right calf.
(4) Correct walking pattern.
(5) Increase muscle tolerance – thereby achieving client's goal of walking in Tibet.
Plan: (1) Soak leg in warm water to restore skin condition, and massage with warm oil. (2) Active exercises with gentle passive stretching at extremes of range. (3) Progress to weight-bearing quickly. (4) Hydrotherapy for walking practice in the pool – water will support yet provide ideal resistance therefore strengthening muscles. (5) Progress to fitness class in gymnasium.
Attendance: Daily for one week. Then three times per week for two weeks. Reduce to twice a week for two weeks when required.
A full recovery is anticipated.

Communication

It requires considerable skill and experience to be able to gain all the relevant information. It has to be appreciated that there is a time factor on both sides, and some clients find it difficult to answer questions in a clinical setting and are confused because they may have been asked similar questions by their GP, or the practice nurse. **Communication skills** are of the utmost importance. To be able to prescribe any form of treatment it is important to find out with a degree of accuracy what is wrong. X-rays, blood tests and pathology reports do not always reveal the whole story.

Practice point

As a support worker who has regular contact with clients, you must:
▷ Encourage the client to have confidence in you. – How do you encourage confidence?
▷ Have the ability to ask the right questions. – Do you always ask open questions?
▷ Be a good listener. – Why is it important to be a good listener?
▷ Have the ability to "read between the lines".
You can refer to Chapter 5, 4 and 6 if you need to remind yourself of the essentials of good communication.

Think about
Think about how you might describe a symptom such as pain or discomfort. (More information on pain is given in Chapter 16.)

Whilst some clients exaggerate when describing their symptoms, others are reluctant to divulge their problems, being shy or stoic and not wishing to "waste your time". Elderly people who may live alone or have low self-esteem often find the whole experience of someone being interested in them and caring for them a very emotional one, and this very fact starts the healing process.

Point to remember

You cannot care without communication.

So communicate with care.

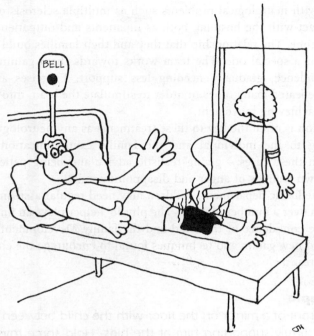

JUST RING THE BELL IF YOUR KNEE GETS TOO HOT MR SMITH
BUT I CAN'T REA..... DON'T WORRY I'LL COME IMMEDIATELY.

The role of the support worker

Just as the physiotherapist is to be found in a variety of settings, then in any of these, the support worker or physio' helper is to be found there too, extending the role of the team. Having chosen to work in a particular specialty, the helper will receive individual training from the physiotherapist and subsequently have his or her own workload. The following points may be useful as a description of this role:

1. To assist the physiotherapist and work under his or her supervision.

2. To work with clients in groups or individually.

3. To be familiar with the working environment and be able to prepare specific treatments.

4. To be familiar with the various items of equipment and ensure that they are maintained in a clean and safe condition.

5. To be able to record accurately details of client treatments.

Safety is given the highest priority. Anything of potential danger to clients or colleagues, whilst being everyone's responsibility, is often specifically noted by helpers – for example, water on the floor from an ice-pack could cause someone to slip if not dried immediately.

Responding to a bell quickly, where a client indicates that a heat treatment is uncomfortably warm, is vital.

Clients with neurological problems such as multiple sclerosis or stroke are often in contact with the hospital, both as inpatients and outpatients, for some considerable time. The relationship that they and their families build up with the physio' dept is a special one. The team works towards them gaining more and more independence, gradually needing less support. Exercises and postural patterns are repeated many times in order to stimulate the brain into recognizing new ways of achieving movement.

Motivation is often the key to these treatments as any neurological problem is devastating to the individual and the family. Communication is of vital importance in these cases – giving realistic advice and being patient with the individual's own feelings of anger and disappointment.

In the paediatric department, children may need regular assessment and are therefore seen over a number of years. The physio' helper plays an important part in gaining the confidence of the child and the family. Development is carefully monitored and new games and techniques found to encourage the child to adopt correct postures.

Example

Sit in front of a mirror on the floor with the child between your knees, firmly supporting him at the hips. Hold some toys just out of reach and encourage the child to stretch and grasp the toys. This encourages him to use his trunk muscles to maintain his balance. You can see just how far to go by looking in the mirror and judging the distances.

On the orthopaedic ward the helper will assist in mobilizing the patient for the first time following surgery. This may entail exercises in bed, or getting the client up on their feet for the first time following a hip replacement. It may also be the helper's responsibility to supply clean, safe walking aids from the department to the client and to know when to progress, giving more responsibility to the client.

In the gymnasium the helper can oversee the exercise regimes of clients who are in the later stages of their rehabilitation. It is all part of the journey to recovery, independence and home.

The physio' helper is indispensible to the running of an efficient department. These posts are increasingly in demand as we look at different ways of utilizing staff to maximum benefit.

Points to remember

- The rehabilitation team has always been the bridge between hospital and home.
- The physiotherapy support worker plays an important part

in the process of recuperation and return to normal function of the client.

■ The support worker's contribution is being recognized as increasingly important as we strive to offer a high-quality dynamic service to a discerning and empowered general public. The support worker thus has an assured future in the rehabilitation department of the year 2000 and beyond.

Further reading

Cartwright (1964), Human Relationships in Hospital Care (Routledge & Kegan Paul).

Calman (1987), Health and Illness – The Lay Perspective (Tavistock).

Hargreaves (1987), "The relevance of non-verbal skills in physiotherapy", Physiotherapy, vol. 73, pages 685–688.

16 | Pain and its management

Fiona Evard

The relief of pain and suffering is one of the most important objectives of health care. Pain is acknowledged to have physiological, psychological and sociological aspects, but it is only within the past 30 years that extensive research into pain processes has produced a greater understanding of pain and – through this understanding – more effective methods of control.

Traditionally, health care workers have had a tendency to hesitate in acknowledging that their clients experience pain, because they have often been at a loss to know how best to offer effective treatment.

This chapter does not intend to be comprehensive but aims to give the support worker an understanding of the complexities of pain processes and how pain can affect individuals.

The support worker's key skill in helping the client in pain is good communication – in particular being able to identify non-verbal cues from clients, and accurate reporting to other members of the health care team. Effective communication and the development of a positive relationship with the client can affect the client's response to pain relief.

The key issues of this chapter are:
- The physiology of pain
- The experience of pain
- Pain and behaviour
- Pain relief

The physiology of pain

Pain is a curious and fascinating concept. Nearly everyone has experienced it; indeed being unable to experience pain is potentially dangerous. Acute pain provides a warning that all is not well and that we need to take some form of action, such as removing the source of the pain or seeking help. **Chronic pain** ceases to have this sort of meaning, but its very persistence has an effect on an individual's whole life and personality.

Pain is a sensation which we generally do not like. As children we learn

This chapter addresses endorsement unit Z19.

about what causes pain, and about how we should respond to it. Culture plays a role in our responses. In this country the tradition has been that men should not cry nor show their emotions, no matter how much pain they are enduring. In some European countries women giving birth are encouraged to make as much noise as possible, and in the Middle East funerals are held amidst the high-pitched wailing of the mourners who are expressing their emotional pain. Who is to say which response is the "healthiest"?

How do we describe pain?

There are hundreds of words to describe pain.

However a person describes pain, their experience of it is unique to them. The sensation of pain is **subjective** and cannot be measured by anyone else except the person who feels it.

> ### Point to remember
>
> "Pain is whatever the experiencing person says it is, existing whenever the experiencing person says it does" (McCaffery, M. 1968 cited in McCaffery and Beebe, 1989)

So, what is this sensation that can strike and leave you gasping with its intensity, or drag on for days, weeks or months and make you feel vulnerable and "under par"?

Imagine a particularly nasty sensation like crushing or burning. There is a

Think about

How many words can you think of to describe pain? A few examples are throbbing, stabbing, burning, aching, intense.

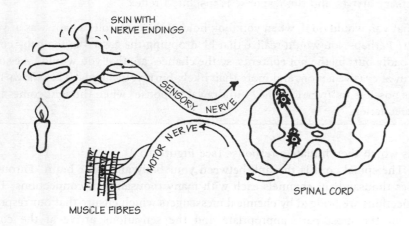

SKIN WITH NERVE ENDINGS

SENSORY NERVE

MOTOR NERVE

SPINAL CORD

MUSCLE FIBRES

THE PAIN REFLEXES INITIATED BY TOUCHING THE HOT CANDLE ARE TRANSMITTED TO THE SPINAL CORD WHICH IN TURN RESULTS IN THE CONTRACTION OF MANY MUSCLES IN THE HAND, ARM AND SHOULDER. THE HAND IS QUICKLY REMOVED. THIS TAKES PLACE SO QUICKLY, THE RESPONSE MAY HAVE OCCURRED SIMULTANEOUSLY WITH THE PERCEPTION OF THE PAIN IN THE BRAIN.

Figure 16.1   A reflex arc

system in the body devoted to the transmission of these unpleasant messages, called the **nociceptive system**, from the Latin word *nocere* meaning to hurt and *capere* meaning to take. It is a very efficient system and once an injured site is identified a number of things happen in a fraction of a second (see Figure 16.1). The message travels from the site of the injury towards the spine, then up the **spinal cord** via specific pathways towards the nerve centre, the **brain**. The brain interprets these messages, makes a response and sends a message back down the spinal cord pathway to the appropriate **muscles**, which will react.

What sensations were you aware of the last time you were under pressure (e.g. taking an exam, driving test or interview)? Did you experience any of the following: dry mouth, butterflies in the stomach, increased perspiration or frequency of urination? These are physical responses to stressful thoughts. Similar sensations may occur following trauma or pain and would then be described as "shock". Fainting may also occur. All these symptoms are initiated by the brain.

When the pain sensations reach the brain, they are interpreted by specific

---

Think about

You have picked up a casserole dish which has just come out of the oven. What happens?

Your immediate response would be to drop it, or have a "withdrawal" response. That is, you would remove your hands from the source of the pain.

This response is automatic: your brain doesn't have time to "think", the message arrives and the response is instant, a reflex.

What you would do if, when you took hold of the casserole, a baby was at your feet? Perhaps you would realize that by dropping the casserole the baby could be badly hurt by the hot contents, so the chances are that you would take some form of evasive action, and more than likely burn your hands! This shows that it is possible to "override" the "withdrawal response" when thought comes into the equation.

---

areas which then initiate a response (see Figure 16.2).

The spinal cord is the link between your body and your brain. Through it passes thousands of channels each with many thousands of connections. These connections are bridged by chemical messengers which ensure that our responses are, for the most part, appropriate and the sensations arrive at the correct destinations.

There are certain occasions when we may want to block the transmission of pain messages, and there are cells known as T cells which seem to be important in initiating this blocking or gating mechanism.

Think about

Have you been in any situation where you were hurt but did not become aware of the injury until some time later?

Example

In the last two minutes of play, in an important football match, the score is 1–1. The centre forward is taking the ball unchal-

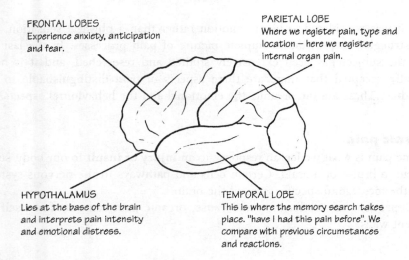

FRONTAL LOBES
Experience anxiety, anticipation and fear.

PARIETAL LOBE
Where we register pain, type and location – here we register internal organ pain.

HYPOTHALAMUS
Lies at the base of the brain and interprets pain intensity and emotional distress.

TEMPORAL LOBE
This is where the memory search takes place. "have I had this pain before". We compare with previous circumstances and reactions.

Figure 16.2   The lobes of the cerebrum (brain)

lenged towards the goal, when suddenly his feet are kicked away from under him as he is viciously tackled, but he can still see the ball within easy reach. He gets up, gains control of the ball and kicks it into goal. The referee blows the final whistle and the cup is theirs! Suddenly the centre forward finds he cannot walk, and investigation reveals he has an open fracture of his shin bone. Obviously this was caused by the tackle, but the excitement masked the pain so that he didn't feel anything such was his involvement in the game.

This is not an uncommon phenomenon. There have been many stories of heroic acts when the hero only noticed his or her own predicament once everyone else was safe. This shows the effectiveness of the blocking mechanism and the powerful effect that *distraction* can have. The phenomenon can be used to advantage – **distraction therapy** can help people to cope more effectively with pain and is mentioned again later in this chapter.

In addition, there are areas of the brain and spinal cord which produce substances called *endorphins* and *enkephalins*. These substances have a morphine-like action which act as the body's internal pain-relieving system, but more research is needed into exactly how these substances are produced.

The experience of pain

Pain is a universal human experience and is the most frequent reason for an individual to seek medical help. In whatever setting you are working you will care for people who have pain. It is therefore important that you are aware of how individuals react to pain and how you can help them.

The very word "pain" is difficult to define, and since the time of Aristotle,

Think about
If you did not feel pain, how might you be at risk?

when it was considered to be an emotion rather than a physical sensation, we have struggled to provide a complete picture of pain processes. In the last 30 years the subject has been extensively studied and researched, and it is now generally accepted that there are three aspects of pain distinguishable to an individual. These are the organic, the emotional and the behavioural aspects.

Organic pain

Organic pain is what we feel in response to an **injury** or **insult** to our body, such as a cut, a bruise or a scald. Certain cells and pathways in the nervous system carry the message to specific areas of the brain.

Dependent on the location and cause, organic pain can manifest itself in different ways:

- *Superficial pain* describes that felt in the skin. The cause is usually due to heat, pressure, puncture or cold.
- *Deep pain* describes that felt in the deep structures of the body, such as muscles or joints. It is sometimes described as "dull" or "gnawing", with a tendency to be longer lasting. It can be affected by activity or body position.
- *Visceral pain* originates from internal organs, and the nature of the pain alters according to the organ affected.
- *Referred pain* is more of a "travelling" pain. Although it originates at a specific point it moves along the nerve pathway. It may be caused by inflammation at the **nerve root**, and the pain is then felt all along the length of the particular nerve and the structures through which it passes. For example, in sciatica, from some untoward occurrence in the region of the lower back there is damage to the nerve root as it arises from the spinal cord, and pain is felt down the length of the back of the leg.
- *Neuralgic pain* may be slightly different in that the actual nervous system itself is the subject of the damage, inflammation or infection. Shingles is a common example of this and is the cause of intense pain.
- *Phantom limb* pain is the strangest phenomenon. Excruciating pain is felt in a "limb" which has been amputated. People experiencing such pain can describe the exact sensations and pinpoint the area of the missing limb that is responsible. The remaining nerves continue to transmit and interpret the sensations with accuracy.

Thing about
When did you last experience pain? Which one of the above categories did it come under?

Emotional aspects of pain

Figure 16.3 illustrates how pain, emotion and tension are so closely linked that it can be difficult to distinguish where one stops and another begins. Look at the factors affecting emotion and consider how they may alter the way you feel on a good day or on a bad day.

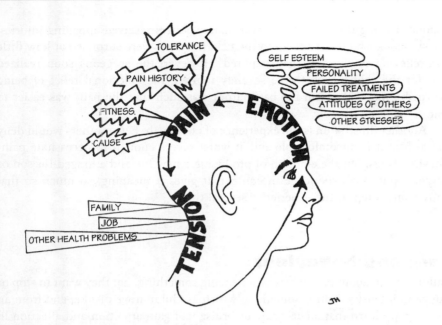

Figure 16.3 Emotional aspects of pain

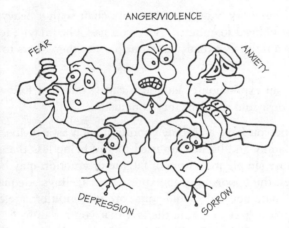

Emotional responses usually accompany pain. They could be anger, fear, sorrow, depression, aggressiveness or violence.

Anxiety and fear may be associated with brief but acute pain, whilst depression and anger are common in those who are suffering from long-term pain caused by a chronic condition. Chronic pain can also create feelings of fatigue and exhaustion, which in turn will have an effect on a person's ability to continue with their normal daily activities. Anxiety and depression make pain difficult to cope with and can alter an individual's character. Partners and carers will also be affected by these emotional changes and relationships can become strained. This in turn creates more tension and so the cycle continues.

The consequences of illness, injury or pain play an important part in how we respond. During the First World War many soldiers received appalling injuries. The surgeons who treated them in the field hospitals were surprised at how little pain-relieving medication they required. However, the surgeons soon realized that, for the soldiers who were severely injured, the emotional relief of being returned home away from the battle front was such that the pain was easier to bear.

Another illustration is the experience of childbirth. Few mothers would deny that at best it is uncomfortable and at worst severe enough to necessitate pain-relieving drugs; but the emotion of producing a new life and a longed-for son or daughter puts the experience in context. It gives it meaning, so much so that many women repeat the experience several times!

Pain and behaviour

Children learn about pain when experiencing something that they want to stop or reduce in intensity. Pain is something which as children we dislike, and from an early age we learn that a cut, graze or bruise will gain attention and affection in terms of reassurance from a parent or adult. Most children will at times seek this

> **Think about**
>
> Arriving home from work, you flop down in a chair with a heavy sigh. Your partner is almost obliged to enquire "Have you had a bad day?", to which you respond "Yes I'm absolutely exhausted". Your partner then offers to make you a cup of tea.
>
> All very normal: an expression of fatigue, a caring question followed with a satisfactory response and a satisfactory conclusion.
>
> However, imagine you have a chronic condition such as arthritis, asthma or migraine. Your family and friends are used to you being less than 100% on occasion and those simple indicators of fatigue or emotion may be ignored. You are not given the opportunity to express your feelings adequately. The people around you do not understand your chronic condition, are embarrassed by it and believe it is best to ignore the fact that you are unwell.

attention by exaggerating or prolonging their symptoms. In later life we use this to a lesser or greater extent.

In such situations pain behaviour may become exaggerated in an attempt to gain a caring response, and as care workers we do sometimes reinforce this in the way we react to clients. When caring for the chronically ill we are more likely to ask "Where have you been feeling the pain?", rather than "What have you achieved this week?" Equally we might say "What a shame you couldn't walk all the way", instead of "Fantastic, you walked 400 yards."

Remember that pain which is openly expressed is easier to deal with than pain which is suppressed by depression, low self-esteem or psychological trauma.

The latter in particular needs specialist help but can respond well. The following example will illustrate this.

Example

A 42-year-old man had been off work for 10 months with back pain following a fall. He had been examined by a number of health professionals but was still in a lot of pain and unable to do much for himself. He was particularly angry with his own doctor and with psychiatrists. On one of his visits he spoke of the traumatic death of his fiance 15 years previously. He had told no-one of her death, only that the engagement was off. Soon after this he emigrated, married and established a family. The long sick leave following his fall had given him a lot of time to himself and his repressed grief manifested itself in anger and depression. After a few sessions of counselling and psycho-therapy he was able to return to work. The pain and grief had been separated and he was then able to take control of his life. The back pain responded very well to treatment.

It is perhaps all too easy to view a condition or diagnosis before recognizing the *person* behind it. From this example we can see that pain is a complex emotion, expressed in a variety of ways, sometimes after years of lying dormant.

Pain and the response to it is complex, but as a health care worker you must be sensitive to its complexities and respect the individual's right to express pain in any way they can. Just as the client has a right to express pain in their own way, the client also has rights in terms of pain relief.

Pain relief and the client's rights

McCaffery and Beebe (1989) state that pain control:

- is a legitimate therapeutic goal
- contributes significantly to the client's physical and emotional well-being
- ranks high as a priority of client care
- is client-controlled.

The client has a right:

- to decide the duration and intensity of pain he or she is willing to endure or tolerate
- to be informed of all possible methods of pain relief along with the favourable and unfavourable consequences as well as the controversial aspects
- to choose which pain control method he or she wishes to try
- to choose to live with or without pain

Everyone who is involved with caring for a client in pain has an important role, although responsibility for choice, timing and administration of pain-relieving methods lie with the health care professionals.

The support worker's role is in understanding how damaging pain can be to the client's self-image and self-esteem, and to support the professional in establishing a treatment alliance which will give the client a feeling of being more in control.

Essential to any form of pain therapy is accurate **assessment** of the client and his or her pain. Remember that pain is what the client says it is, and to help in assessing the degree and location of pain an assessment tool can be used. It may be in the form of a simple visual scale:

No pain ———————————————————— **worst pain imaginable**

The client marks on the scale the degree of pain felt.

You should be alert to the fact that children may have difficulty in identifying the exact location of their pain, and frequently a "sore tummy" can mean pain anywhere but in the tummy.

Once the client's pain has been assessed accurately, a variety of pain-relieving methods may be considered.

Pharmacological control

A wide variety of drugs can help to relieve pain. They range from mild analgesics, to anti-inflammatory drugs, to strong narcotic drugs. The choice of drug and its method of administration are dependent on the needs of the individual client.

In many acute care settings, clients are now able to control their own pain relief through "patient controlled analgesia systems". It is interesting to note that clients who can control their own analgesia usually need less.

Example

We rejoin our footballer from earlier in this chapter, in the casualty department. He is about to be X-rayed and operated on, and is going to be experiencing many of the sensations on our original list. But pain is the most immediate, and until it is controlled it will govern every other response, and prevent progress.

In his case, medication is necessary to control these unpleasant sensations. Once the fracture is healing and his rehabilitation programme is under way, there are other means to control the pain he will undoubtedly feel as he regains the range of movement in his knee and ankle, and builds up the muscles that have wasted since the original accident. The therapist will give him confidence, but be sensitive to his anxieties, whilst motivating him to the fullest possible recovery.

Transcutaneous electrical nerve stimulation (TENS)

The idea of electrical stimulation for pain relief is not new. Some 2000 years ago the Roman physician Scribonius Largus applied electric eels to haemorrhoids, arthritis, headaches and the feet of gout sufferers!

The modern apparatus is a compact battery-operated machine with small electrodes which are placed around the site of the pain. The mild stimulation delivered helps to confuse the pain nerve endings and brings relief.

TENS can be used to treat acute pain, chronic pain, postoperative pain and discomfort during the first stage of labour.

Nerve block

Nerve block can give effective pain relief in a high proportion of clients who have nerve irritation or invasion. The nerve pathway is interrupted either by surgery or by means of injecting a drug into a specific site.

A well-known type of nerve block is the epidural anaesthetic which is frequently used to provide pain relief for women in labour.

Distraction and diversion

Distraction from pain can be defined as focusing attention on stimuli other than the pain sensation. It should be remembered that distraction does not make the pain disappear but does make it more bearable.

Depending on the nature of the illness and on the individual, some diversion which is acceptable to the client provides distraction that may reduce his concentration on the pain. Talking with others, reading, watching television or guided imagery may focus the client's thoughts on more pleasant sensations.

Psychotherapy

Relaxation causes physiological responses which include reduction in heart rate, respiration and muscle tension. Many people mistakenly believe that flopping down in front of the television is being relaxed, but true relaxation is only achieved through learned techniques and conscious effort.

For the client with pain, learning to relax using self-hypnosis or other methods can reduce tension, aid sleep, increase self-confidence and promote self-control.

Massage and slow rhythmic deep breathing

These techniques complement some of the others in aiming to relax the client and teach ways of gaining and maintaining control over pain.

Complementary therapies

A variety of so-called "complementary therapies" are gaining recognition and being more widely used within care settings. They help to promote a holistic approach to the management of acute and chronic pain.

Acupuncture is the ancient Chinese practice of inserting fine needles into specific points along the "meridians" of the body to relieve the discomfort associated with painful disorders, to induce anaesthesia and for preventative and therapeutic purposes.

Aromatherapy is the use of essential oils which have been extracted from plants. The oils are used in the treatment of medical conditions or as relaxing agents.

Practice point
Try and find out more about complementary therapies to enable you to provide accurate information to your clients.

Homeopathy is a system of therapeutics founded by Samual Hahnemann (1755–1843) in which diseases are treated by drugs that are capable of producing in healthy persons symptoms like those of the disease to be treated, the drug being administered in minute doses.

Osteopathy is a system of therapy utilizing generally accepted methods of diagnosis, and emphasizing the importance of normal body mechanics and manipulative methods of detecting and correcting faulty structure.

Reflexology is a therapy based on the belief that the body's natural healing mechanisms can be enhanced by the application of pressure to certain areas of the feet and hands. These areas are said to be connected to different parts of the body by a flow of energy. The term "reflex" refers to the "reflection" of organs on to the skin's surface.

Fundamental to all these therapies is the effective use of communication skills. Talking with and actively listening to your client will go a long way to reducing anxiety, relieving tension and lessening pain. Providing the client with information and helping the client to participate in management of their pain is also very important.

Point to remember
Managing pain is much more than just treating the initial problem. As a health care worker you need to understand and be sensitive to the needs of the individual and the effect their injury or illness has had upon them.

Further reading

McCaffery and Beebe (1989), Clinical Manual for Nursing Practice (Mosby). This book provides comprehensive information on aspects of pain and is of value to professional and non-professional carers.

Jacques (1994), "The physiology of pain", British Journal of Nursing, vol. 3.

Nursing Times Special Issue (autumn 1993), "Complementary therapy". A valuable resource for all carers, which explains a range of complementary therapies.

REFERENCES

McCaffery, M. and Beebe, A. (1989). *Clinical Manual for Nursing Practice* (Mosby).

Promotion of continence

17

Stephanie Pye

Incontinence is a very common problem. One in four women and one in ten men experience some urinary incontinence at some stage in their lives (Thomas et al. 1980). It is therefore not surprising that most people will know someone who experiences incontinence.

Incontinence may be cured by effective treatment or improved by effective management, thereby improving the quality of a person's life.

There is a great deal of stigma associated with incontinence, and people are frequently too embarrassed even to discuss the subject. As a support worker you have an important role in promoting continence and effectively managing incontinence.

The key issues of this chapter are:
- Reasons for urinary incontinence
- Attitudes and stigma surrounding incontinence
- How to promote continence
- Treatments for incontinence
- Effective management of incontinence.

What is urinary incontinence?

Many people believe that incontinence is the loss of a large amount of urine, but the following definition shows that the amount of urine loss is only part of the problem:

‘*(Urinary incontinence is) involuntary excretion or leakage of urine in an inappropriate place or at inappropriate times twice or more per month, regardless of the quantity of urine lost*’

Thomas et al. (1980)

This chapter links with the O Unit, Z4, Y2, U4 and endorsement unit Z12.

The image of continence has changed over the years and what is considered normal in one culture may be very different from another. It was only in the nineteenth century that toilets were designed and used – before that people used the gutters in the street and the rich reserved their cellars for the purpose. In France it is perfectly acceptable for men to pass urine openly by the side of a main road, while the average British male disappears behind a tree 25 yards away from the road edge!

Who is incontinent?

A large-scale study showed that about 25% of women and 10% of men suffered from urinary incontinence on two or more occasions per month, although the majority did not seek any help. The incidence increases considerably in men over the age of 65 years, while in women it occurs more evenly across the age range.

1:4 WOMEN

1:10 MEN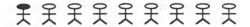

The higher incidence of stress incontinence in women may be attributed to childbirth and hormonal changes after the menopause.

Although the study took place in this country some time ago, it is still frequently quoted (Thomas et al. 1980).

The number of incontinent clients in long-stay elderly wards is high, but equally it is worth noting that a high proportion of clients in acute care settings are also incontinent.

What is "normal"?

We are all born "incontinent". The achievement of continence is a gradual process acquired through the maturation of the central nervous system and by teaching the child to use a toilet. The age at which this is achieved varies considerably. However, most children are reliably dry during the day by the time they start school, but one in six children at 5 years of age will still be wetting the bed at night (Blackwell 1989).

- Most adults empty their bladder between three and six times in a 24-hour period.
- Most adult bladders hold between 400 and 600 millilitres of urine, but most people will pass urine before reaching the full capacity.
- Most people will have a warning signal before they pass urine. For example, if you are driving along the motorway you can hold on until it is convenient to stop.

Think about
Think about what issues or factors are important in each situation.

Factors affecting the ability to be continent

The balance between continence and incontinence may be altered by one or more of the four factors featured in Figure 17.1, or by an underlying bladder problem which may be temporary or permanent.

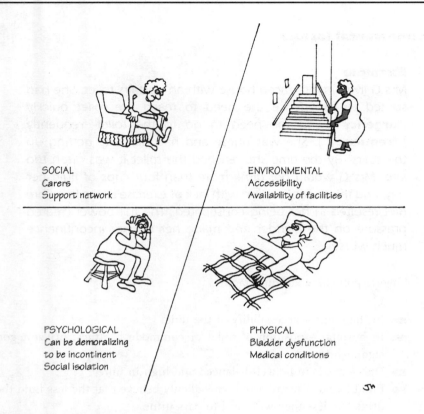

Figure 17.1   Factors affecting continence

Social factors

Example

A district nurse was visiting Mrs A, an 80-year-old lady who lived with her 78-year-old brother. She had chronic arthritis which restricted her mobility. She spent most of the day sitting in an armchair in the front room. She could reach the downstairs toilet but needed help to get out of the chair. Her brother spent most of the day outside the home doing his own activities and refused to help.

Mrs A was incontinent. This was not due to a lack of bladder control but because she did not have the help she needed to reach the toilet.

Point to remember

Carers and support networks are important factors in the ability to be continent.

Environmental factors

Example
Mrs G lived in a terraced house with an upstairs toilet. She had started to experience the need to reach the toilet quickly ("**urgency**") and the need to go to the toilet frequently ("**frequency**"). She was obese and had difficulty getting up the stairs. By the time she reached the toilet it was often too late. Mrs G would not drink more than four cups of fluid per day, and this in conjunction with lack of exercise and a low-fibre diet resulted in her being constipated. The full bowel created pressure on the bladder and made her urinary incontinence much worse.

The following points are all important:

- In the home – accessibility of the toilet
- In hospital – position of toilet or commode facilities; privacy; good signposting
- Diet – needs to be well-balanced and high in fibre
- Fluid intake – many people mistakenly believe that the less fluid they drink the less they will need to pass urine.

Physical factors
There are many conditions which either have a direct effect on bladder function, affect mobility, or exacerbate existing incontinence. Such conditions include diabetes, stroke ("cerebral vascular accident") and multiple sclerosis. A client who has had a stroke, for example, may have impairment of bladder function, but this is compounded by the difficulty with balance and walking. Poor eyesight and reduced dexterity can also make it difficult to undo clothes in time.

Constipation or faecal impaction will cause pressure on the bladder and create problems. Urinary tract infections will have an adverse effect on bladder function.

Point to remember
Be alert to the medical diagnosis of the underlying problem.

Psychological factors
A person who is suffering from depression or who is lacking in motivation may not be particularly interested in remaining continent.

For those who are incontinent the effect has been described by some sufferers as "depressing, distressing and totally demoralizing".

Many people reduce their outside activities and gradually become more and more socially isolated. Others completely deny their incontinence because of the stigma and the association with childhood.

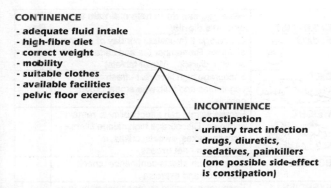

Figure 17.2   The fine balance between continence and incontinence

Point to remember

Incontinence has a major impact on the way people see and feel about themselves.

Attitudes and taboos surrounding incontinence

Until very recently, incontinence was a subject rarely discussed. It was considered a taboo subject. This situation was not helped by dictionary definitions of the word, which include "lack of restraint" and "lewdness".

People frequently comment that their incontinence makes them feel dirty and unacceptable, which in turn causes embarrassment. This embarrassment can become even more acute when a person needs carers to help deal with it.

There is a misconception that incontinence and increasing age go hand in hand, people often saying "It's just my age" or "What do you expect at 75 years old!". There are also many women who mistakenly believe that incontinence is to be expected following childbirth. These beliefs and misconceptions are now being discussed much more openly. The press and media are prepared to feature articles and discussions on incontinence, a condition which affects more than three million people.

Support workers have an important role in enabling people to express their fears and feelings about their incontinence and to provide accurate and reliable information to clients and their carers.

Think about

How do you feel about caring for someone who is incontinent? You may well think "It's just part of the job."

But how would you feel if you were caring for a relative who was incontinent? A daughter caring for her mother may not be seen as posing a problem, but how difficult would it be for a son to care for his incontinent mother, or for a daughter to put a sheath on her father to manage his incontinence better?

CHECKLIST	What **you** can do to help maintain a person's dignity	Tick Box
FLUIDS 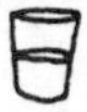	Encourage 6 (mugsize) per day of a variety of drinks. Remember tea and coffee may act as a diuretic. (Water tablets)	
DIET 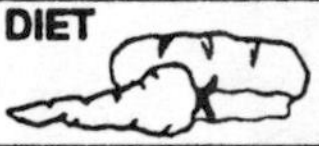	Encourage high fibre diet - fresh vegetables and fruit, wholemeal bread, cereals	
WEIGHT 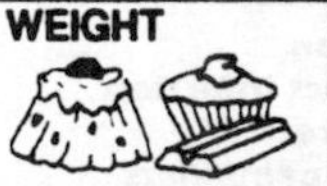	Excess weight can affect ability to remain continent. Discourage high calorie fillers - biscuits, cakes, sweets, crisps, ie moderation - not excess	
BOWELS	Constipation affects continence, check diet, fluids and exercise	
EXERCISE 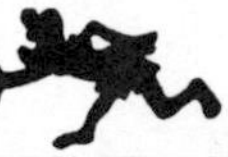	Encourage mobility as far as possible, ie a short walk round the home is better than none at all. Everybody can benefit from pelvic floor exercises	
MOBILITY 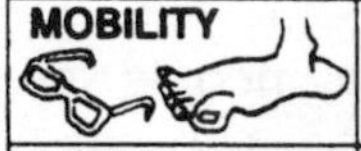	Does the lady/gentleman need to see chiropodist/optician/occupational therapist?	
BATH/ HYGIENE 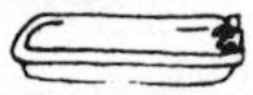	Don't use Dettol/Savlon in baths Regular showers/baths reduce the risk of urinary tract infection plus a high fluid intake	
CLOTHES 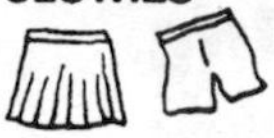	Are these easy to manage? Female - eg 'A' line skirts, french knickers Male - velcro on trousers, long fly openings, boxer shorts	
ENVIRONMENT 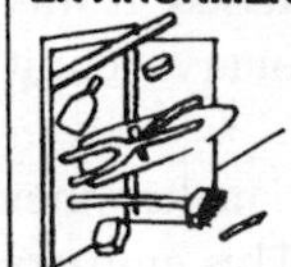	Do they get much warning before passing urine? - if not .. Does the person need to sit closer to the toilet? Are the toilets accessible - is there a clear access? Do you need adaptations - handrails etc	

Figure 17.3   Advice to offer to clients

Promotion of continence

The support worker is part of the care team and as such has an important role in the promotion of continence. The chart in Figure 17.3 illustrates what advice you can offer to your clients.

It is important to remember that an assessment of the client's condition and circumstances must be carried out to identify the problem and to discuss possible solutions. For a full nursing continence assessment, refer to the senior nurse or district nursing sister.

Following assessment the client may be referred to the GP for medical investigations, the continence advisor for specialised treatment, advice on aids, pads, sheaths etc., or to the physiotherapist for pelvic floor exercises.

Types of bladder dysfunction

This part of the chapter will explain in some detail types of bladder dysfunction and the interventions that can be used to treat and/or improve the condition.

Practice points

▶ Is there a continence advisor in your area? Do you know how, where and when to contact him/ her?

▶ Are there any continence clinics held locally, either in the health centre or hospital?

▶ Is there a Health Promotion Unit in your area where you can obtain information leaflets?

Table 17.1   Four types of bladder dysfunction

	Symptoms	Nursing intervention
Detrusor instability ("unstable bladder")	Urgency; urge incontinence; frequency; nocturnal enuresis; nocturia	Bladder retraining and possibly anti-cholinergic drugs
Stress incontinence	Leakage on exertion (e.g. coughing, sneezing, running)	Pelvic floor exercises
Outflow obstruction	Dribbling; voiding difficult	Intermittent self-catheterization
Atonic bladder	Overflow incontinence	instruction in voiding technique

There are four main types of bladder dysfunction, outlined in Table 17.1. It is important to have a knowledge of these to aid understanding of the complex nature of incontinence and to highlight the need for accurate assessment.

Detrusor instability

Detrusor instability, or "unstable bladder", occurs because of involuntary bladder muscle contractions while the bladder is filling with urine, resulting in the bladder emptying. The person will recognize the need to pass urine but may not be able to reach the toilet in time. For people with restricted mobility the reduced warning time can make life very difficult indeed.

To help overcome this problem, a bladder retraining programme can be introduced which aims to gradually increase the time between voiding. The programme needs to be systematic and involves maintaining a record of when, where and how urine was passed.

As it can be very difficult to deliberately wait to use the toilet, some people find it easier to use a form of distraction. One client known to the author used to sew another 100 stitches in her tapestry, to help increase the time between visits to the toilet.

Some of the possible causes of detrusor instability include stroke, multiple sclerosis, diabetes. In some cases there is no apparent cause.

It is important to encourage people to keep an accurate record of when, where and how urine was passed. If your client is unable to do this you must maintain a record for them. Figure 17.4 illustrates a chart which could be used by both you and your clients.

Stress incontinence

Stress incontinence is the symptom of leaking urine during physical exertion. It may occur during very active exercise such as aerobics, or simply by coughing and sneezing. Obesity and smoking with a chronic cough exacerbates this type of

Name...

Week Commencing:...

Please tick in left column each time urine is passed and record volume if possible.
Please write 'D' 'C' or 'S' in right column each time you are wet.
'D'=damp 'C'=clothes wet 'S'=soaked ie clothes and furniture wet.

	Monday		Tuesday		Wednesday		Thursday		Friday		Saturday		Sunday	
6am														
.15														
.30														
.45														
7am														
.15														
.30														
.45														
8am														
.15														
.30														
.45														
9am														
.15														
.30														
.45														
10am														
.15														
.30														
.45														
11am														
.15														
.30														
.45														
12noon														
.15														
.30														
.45														
1pm														
.15														
.30														
.45														
2pm														

Figure 17.4   A baseline urine chart

incontinence. Encouraging clients to reduce weight and to stop smoking will help.

Stress incontinence is more common in women, and childbirth is one of the possible causes. Weakening of the pelvic floor muscles is more likely in women who have had a prolonged second stage of labour, had a rapid delivery, or who have had a number of babies in fairly quick succession.

After the menopause, some women may experience stress incontinence due to the alterations in hormone levels. This alteration can result in a dry vagina and sagging of the muscles of the pelvic floor.

Anatomically, women have a much shorter urethra than men and the position of it in relation to other organs makes it more vulnerable to damage.

Depending on the severity of the stress incontinence, pelvic floor exercises can be very helpful. These exercises are taught to women attending antenatal classes, but they should be taught also to young girls before they become pregnant, as part of their health education. As a support worker you have an important role in reinforcing the need to practice pelvic floor exercises. The following is a summary.

> **Practice point**
> Revise or familiarize yourself with the anatomy of male and female pelvic organs.

- Sit, stand or lie, and without tensing the muscles of your legs, buttocks or abdomen, tighten the ring of muscle around the anus, imagining that you are trying to control the passing of a stool. This will help you identify the back part of the pelvic floor.
- When you are passing urine, try to stop the flow then restart it. Do this for *one day only* to help you become aware of the front muscles of the pelvic floor. Thereafter you could do this as a "check" every week on just one occasion.
- Working from back to front, tighten the muscles whilst slowly counting to four, then release them. Repeat this six times – twice in the morning, twice in the afternoon and twice in the evening, until you regain control. Then do this twice a day to help maintain control forever. Keep a record of doing the exercises. You can do this exercise anywhere – sitting or standing, whilst watching television or waiting for a bus. There is no need to interrupt your normal daily activity.
- After practising for two or three weeks, you will feel the closure of the front and back passages and a drawing up of the pelvic floor in front. Do not tighten the abdominal, thigh, or buttock muscles, or cross your legs in order to feel the pelvic muscles. Do not worry if you are not successful at once. *Practise and persevere.*

Point to remember
Many women accept stress incontinence as a natural consequence of having children, but they do not have to endure this distressing symptom. You can help them to help themselves by giving them the information they need and supporting them.

Assessment of the severity of the symptom will assist in the choice of treatment. Treatments other than exercises include hormone replacement therapy (HRT) or specialized treatment by the physiotherapist.

The physiotherapist may use vaginal cones or electrical stimulation of specific muscles. Vaginal cones can be used as an assessment tool to establish the condition of pelvic muscles, and as an aid to exercise. The cones are weighted and when one is inserted into the vagina the woman has to contract her pelvic floor muscles to retain it. Initially the lightest cone is used. The aim is to gradually increase the time the cone can be retained (up to 10 minutes twice a day) and then increase the weight of the cone. The cones are not disposable and need to be washed, dried and stored in their case. Each client has her own set of cones.

Faradism and interferential therapy are types of electrical stimulation used by the physiotherapist. Carefully controlled electrical current is passed through electrodes to identified areas of the vagina to stimulate specific pelvic floor muscles to contract more efficiently. This form of treatment may need to be carried out regularly over a period of time.

Outflow obstruction

When there is a hindrance to the outflow of urine, this is described as "outflow obstruction". Possible causes include an enlarged prostate gland or faecal impaction. The treatment involves dealing with the cause of the obstruction.

> **Point to remember**
> It is useful to remember that owing to the anatomical proximity of bladder and bowel, a full or impacted bowel can indirectly cause urinary problems.

Atonic bladder

An atonic bladder is one that does not contract sufficiently to ensure complete bladder emptying. Some of the possible causes include spinal injury, multiple sclerosis or any condition affecting the bladder nerves.

Drug therapy may be useful in helping the bladder to contract. Otherwise, complete emptying can only be obtained through abdominal effort or manual expression.

Passive incontinence

Passive incontinence can occur for any of the reasons described, or for no obvious reason and without any warning. This form of incontinence frequently occurs in clients who are suffering from confusion or dementia, and in those who have learning difficulties.

In many hospitals and care settings the practice of routine toileting of clients is still carried out, regardless of whether or not the clients wish to or have a need to empty their bladder. This is a task-orientated approach to care and does not take into account the individual needs and requirements of clients. The use of individualized toilet regimes combined with behaviour modification programmes are more effective than routine toileting on a four-hourly basis.

An individual regime involves maintaining a half-hourly check and recording of the moisture content of the client's body-worn pads over a period of three days (day-time only). From these records the senior nurse in charge of the assessment will establish the peak emptying times of the bladder. The client is then assisted to the toilet a quarter of an hour before these peak times and encouraged to void urine. Over a period of time for many people this regime is an effective way of preventing incontinence, maintaining dignity and self-respect.

It is important to recognize each client as an individual and to avoid labelling or passively accepting incontinence in clients who are old, have a mental health problem or learning difficulty. Concentrating on individual needs will take more time, but in the long term the quality of life for the client will improve and there will be greater satisfaction for carers. It will also be less costly on all resources.

> **Practice point**
> If possible, arrange with your supervisor or senior nurse to observe a continence assessment.

Point to remember
Your role in accurately recording information is crucial for accurate planning.

Assessment

Assessment is crucial and requires a multidisciplinary approach. It needs to cover:

- social, physical, environmental and psychological factors.
- a full medical examination by the GP or hospital doctor
- a mid-stream urine specimen (MSU) to exclude urinary tract infection, which can cause frequency by triggering the bladder to empty more frequently
- a rectal examination to exclude constipation
- baseline charting (can *you* remember when you last passed urine?).

The mutlidisciplinary team involved in assessing, promoting, treating and managing incontinence includes the following members:

It is important for all members of the team to record and communicate accurately, and to encourage people not to accept their incontinence passively. They should be helped to overcome their embarrassment over this distressing

- nursing team and support workers
- medical team
- GP
- geriatrician
- urologist
- gynaecologist
- physiotherapist
- occupational therapist
- social worker

problem.

Effective management of incontinence

There is a wide range of options for managing incontinence. They include body-worn pads, male penile sheaths, male appliances, intermittent self-catheterization, and indwelling urinary catheter.

Experience helps not only in selecting the right product for individual clients but also in the correct method of application of the product. Consider the key words in more detail.

- *Acceptability* – Does the client feel happy with the product? Some men, for example, prefer not to use a pad as they consider them to be "only for women".
- *Availability* – Is the product easily available? The products may be available free on the NHS, on prescription or purchased commercially. With certain items there may be a limited choice and a restriction on the amount issued.
- *Effectiveness* – Does the product contain the incontinence effectively without leakage or discomfort?
- *Cost* – The cost of the product is very important. Many health care organizations will offer a limited range and number of pads for example, to people living at home. Within a hospital setting there may also be a limited range of products offered.

More detailed information on all these products is available in the ACA *Directory of Continence and Toileting Aids*.

Body-worn pads

These pads are held in place by mesh pants. The size of the pad denotes what volume of urine it will hold. Extra long pads are available to contain faecal incontinence. Some shaped pads will hold up to 750 millilitres of urine. All-in-one pads are available from baby size to extra-large adult size. "Marsupial pants" are so called because they contain a pouch for the pad.

A major advantage of body-worn pads is that they are relatively easy to apply and this is particularly helpful for carers. In addition they may be supplied by the local health authority or hospital. The disadvantage of body-worn pads relates to the quality of the particular pad. Bulky pads can be uncomfortable and clients may feel that the pad is visible through their clothing.

Penile sheaths

Penile sheaths are available on prescription from the GP. In hospital there may be other brands of sheaths available.

One advantage of the sheath is its acceptability, in particular to men who are accustomed to applying contraceptive sheaths. However, some men with sensitive skin may find that there needs to be a gradual build-up of time spent wearing a sheath.

The disadvantages include a number of common problems which at first may discourage male clients from using them. The application of the sheath requires a degree of dexterity by the man or his carer, and clients who are confused or suffering from dementia will frequently pull the sheath off. There may be some embarrassment on behalf of the client or carer, in particular if a daughter is caring for her father.

One of the most common problems is that the sheath keeps falling off. The penis may be too retracted, a common difficulty in older men. If when a man sits down there is less than one centimetre of penis showing, then it is impossible to fit a sheath properly. A shorter length sheath is available for the man with a short penis.

The sheath may be the wrong size. There is a tendency to fit a smaller size in an attempt to keep it on, but this will only make the client more uncomfortable. When selecting the correct size you should remember to leave a gap of 1–2 centimetres at the top of the glans penis, otherwise the pressure of urinating will force the sheath off.

The sheath may simply not be acceptable, in which case the man will continue to pull it off.

Practice point
Do you know which type of penile sheaths are available in your work area? Have you experienced problems with the application of penile sheaths, and if so how have you managed?

Body-worn appliances

Body-worn appliances are available on prescription, but must be fitted by an expert. The client will need some time to become accustomed to wearing such an appliance. For some men, body-worn appliances are highly acceptable.

They are particularly useful for men who are unable to wear sheaths because of a retracted penis. They are also of value, if the man or his carer has difficulty in fitting a sheath, and they involve less penile contact so reducing embarrassment.

Their main disadvantage is that the appliances need to be well maintained and are not suitable for use during the night.

The client is usually given two appliances: one to wear whilst the other is washed. They need to be changed daily and should be washed in warm soapy water, thoroughly dried, dusted with a small amount of talcum powder and placed in a warm dry place, for example the airing cupboard. If the appliance is cared for in this way it should last for up to 6 months. Once the appliance has been correctly fitted there should be no need to keep undoing the buttons.

Intermittent self-catheterization

The technique of passing a small catheter at regular intervals to empty the bladder has been used for centuries. Initially, small tubes made of bronze were used and, later the Chinese used onion leaves. In the eighteenth century men who had gonococcal urethral strictures used a silver catheter which they kept tucked in their hats. In America during the 1960s the technique was used as a sterile procedure, by carers in spinal injury units, and by the early 1970s the procedure was being used in the UK.

Intermittent self-catheterization is suitable only for clients with certain types of bladder dysfunction, so the client must be assessed and have urodynamic measurements taken.

The advantages of this technique are that it improves the client's quality of life, avoids the need for an indwelling catheter, and keeps the risk of urinary tract

Practice point
Is there a body-worn appliance fitter in your local area?
Are you familiar with how to care for appliances?

Practice point
Have you cared for
someone who has
used self-
catheterization? If not,
try to arrange to meet
someone who does
and to discuss how he
or she feels about
intermittent self-
catheterization.

infections low. In addition the client can retain responsibility and control over their own health and the ability to have a normal sexual relationship. One client with multiple sclerosis who uses this technique said: "It may only be six inches of plastic but it's worth everything to me."

Although age is no barrier the client does need to have a degree of dexterity, and the client's bladder capacity should be more than 100 millilitres.

Indwelling urinary catheters

Indwelling urinary catheters are available on prescription and can be used in a variety of situations. The most common reasons for their use are to drain urine from the bladder before or after an operation, where there is a blockage (e.g. an enlarged prostate), as part of a special investigation, or for the management of long-term incontinence.

Catheters and drainage bags are available in a variety of different sizes and materials, with shorter catheters available for women. It is important to ensure that the correct size and length of catheter is used, and worth remembering that "small is beautiful".

Client assessment is essential to provide the correct option and to maintain client dignity.

Indwelling catheters should be the last choice in the management of incontinence, because:

- one or two out of every five people in hospital will develop a urinary tract infection (Roe 1992)
- many people with long-term catheters experience problems of leakage around the catheter, blockage and not least discomfort and indignity
- for young people with long-term catheters, renal complications become a major cause of morbidity and mortality.

The day-to-day practice of caring for and teaching a client to manage their catheter is crucial in helping to reduce some of these problems. For you as a support worker, taking steps to reduce the risk of infection by complying with all infection control measures is of paramount importance (see also Chapter 12).

Caring for the client with an indwelling catheter

Personal hygiene is important to the client to maintain his or her self-esteem. If the client prefers to have a bath rather than a shower, the drainage bag must be supported, and must be lower than the level of the bladder to allow free drainage of urine. Avoid spiggoting the catheter as each time there is a break in the closed system there is an increased risk of introducing infection.

Care must be taken to ensure the tube does not *kink*, and good-quality leg straps to hold the bag in place will prevent unnecessary and uncomfortable movement of the catheter in the urethra.

When emptying a catheter bag, wear disposable gloves and always wash your

Practice point
What types of
catheters, leg bags,
night drainage bags
and straps are
available in your work
area?

hands before and after handling the bag. The bag should be emptied before it reaches its maximum capacity. However, if the bag is emptied every time there is a small amount of urine in it you are increasing the risk of infection by breaking the closed system unnecessarily. If the bag is too full, then the weight of the bag will pull on the catheter.

Point to remember

Every time the bag is emptied or changed, or a catheter specimen is taken, the system is opened allowing the entry of bacteria.

The client should be encouraged to drink 2.5–3.0 litres of fluid per day (unless the client is on restricted fluid) to keep the urine clear. A high-fibre diet will help prevent constipation and avoid problems in drainage.

For clients who are sexually active, the organization SPOD (Sexual Problems Of the Disabled) will be able to offer sensitive advice and information.

When the client is to be discharged, he or she needs to be given the opportunity to practise self-care of the catheter and to be supported in this for several days prior to going home. Written information should be given to act as a reminder, and arrangements should be made for the district nurse to visit the client as soon as possible after discharge.

Other useful equipment

Non-spill adaptors are placed in urinal bottles to prevent spillage. These are particularly useful for male clients at night.

Plastic coverings can be used to protect pillows, mattresses and duvets, but they can be uncomfortable and hot for the client. They are available from leading chemists.

Points to remember

- Your role is important in reassuring clients that incontinence is not inevitable and that there are ways to treat, improve or manage it effectively.
- Demonstrating a positive attitude is an important step in encouraging people to talk about, accept and deal with this "embarrassing" problem.
- The success of treatment and management also depends on accurate recording, reporting and encouragement by the whole multidisciplinary team.

Practice point
Are there written standards on catheter care in your work area? Is there a leaflet available on catheter care for clients and carers?

Practice Activity
Think about how you have helped someone to manage their incontinence effectively. Share your thoughts and ideas with your colleagues and consider how you might improve your practice.

Glossary

Constipation. The term used to indicate either the infrequent passage of stools (two or less per week) or excessive straining on defaecation.

Detrusor. A general term for a body part (e.g. a muscle that pushes down).

Faecal impaction. Faeces loading in the rectum and/or colon, with a large amount of stool of any consistency.

Frequency. Most people pass urine between three and six times per day. If a person passes urine seven or more times in 24 hours, this would be considered as frequency.

Nocturia. This means rising at night to pass urine.

Nocturnal enuresis. Passing urine whilst asleep.

Stress incontinence. The symptom of leaking urine during physical exertion, such as coughing, laughing or lifting. It may occur only on exercise (e.g. aerobics) or in severe cases with very little movement.

Urgency. Is the symptom of having to rush to pass urine and there may be very little warning (a few minutes only). If the person cannot reach the toilet in time, urge incontinence may result.

Useful addresses

Association for Continence Advice (ACA), The Basement, 2 Doughty Street, London WC1N 2PH (0171 404 6821).

Association to Aid the Sexual and Personal Relationships of People with a Disability (SPOD), 286 Camden Road, London N7 0BJ (0171 607 8851).

Continence Advisory Service (0191 213 0050) between 2pm and 7pm.

Disabled Living Foundation, 380–384 Harrow Road, London W9 2HU (0171 289 6111).

Enuresis Resource and Information Centre (ERIC), 65 St Michael's Hill, Bristol BS2 8DZ (0272 264 920).

Further reading

Bell (1994), Bedwetting – A Guide for Parents (Enuresis Resource and Information Centre).

Feneley and Blanin (1984), Incontinence: Patient Handbook (Churchill Livingstone).

Medill (1991), Try for Dry (Caretaker Ltd, Sherbourne).

Millard, (1987), Overcoming Urinary Incontinence (Thorsons).

Morgan(1988), Help for the Bedwetting Child (Methuen).

Fader and Norton (1994), Caring for Continence – A Care Assistant's Guide (Hawker Publications).

References

Blackwell, C. (1989). *A Guide to Enuresis* (Enuresis Resource and Information Centre).

Norton, C. (1986). *Nursing for Continence* (England Beaconsfield Publishers).

Roe, B. (1992). *Clinical Nursing Practise: The Promotion and Management of Continence* (Prentice Hall).

Thomas, T.M, Plymatt, K.R., Blanin, J. and Meade, T.(1980). "Prevalence of urinary incontinence", *British Medical Journal*, vol. 281, pp. 1243–1245.

APPENDICES

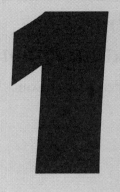

Study skills

(i)

Time management

Aileen Richardson

How often have you asked "Where has my week gone"? On reflection, did you really know where your week had gone? Probably you did not, and certainly not in any detail. It must follow, therefore, that the first step in the management of your time is an **audit** – not merely of the activities you undertake but also of the *time* taken to complete those activities. Since time is precious you should avoid using too much of it in the construction of an elaborate inventory. Keep it simple! Keep it basic!

Your time log

Design a time log. A very simple format will suffice. Sheets of ruled A4 or foolscap, additionally ruled by yourself in three columns headed respectively "Time", "Activity" and "Time taken", will be quite adequate. Over the next seven days make an entry for each activity, as in Figure A1.1.

Analysis

At the end of the week, astonish yourself by noting how much unproductive time has been recorded! How many people do you know who are extremely busy (you never witness an idle moment in their day) but who achieve very little in reality, and whose productivity far from justifies the time expended in the completion of the task in hand? Then ask yourself if your time log seems to point to you being just such a person.

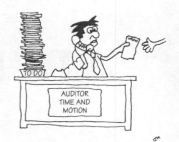

WHAT A GREAT BACKHAND – OH, ER, YES I'LL SEE TO THAT, THANK YOU – ANYWAY I KNEW HE WAS GOING TO WIN AFTER THE FIRST GAME.

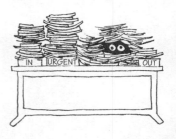

NOW I KNOW THOSE FILES ARE HERE SOMEWHERE

To mention just one or two examples, it is all too easy to spend time chatting over the break about last Saturday's tennis tournament, to do things yourself instead of delegating or sharing tasks (after all, you are not the only person in the organization with a knowledge of the subject), or to be untidy in your work – thereby necessitating a time-consuming search every time you need a document or a piece of equipment.

Time	Activity	Time taken
Mon: 06.30	Get up, have breakfast	1hr
07.00	Walk the dog	10 mins
07.30	Get ready for work	20 mins
08.00–13.00	At work	5hrs
13.30	Walk the dog	15 mins
14.00	Shopping	1hr
15.30	Watch TV/fall asleep	2hrs
17.00	Prepare meal and eat	45 mins
18.30	Phone friend	30 mins
19.00	Iron/watch TV	3hrs
22.00	Let the dog out and prepare for bed	15 mins

Figure A1.1   Time log

Tim is 34, works as a trainee health care assistant and is working towards an NVQ at level 3. His interests include athletics and he supports his local football club. His wife works in an office. He has two sons aged 8 and 10 years.

	Work	Leisure	Home	Study
Monday	7.00am – 4.00pm			Evening study 7pm – 9pm
Tuesday	1.30pm – 9.30pm			10am – 12pm Morning study Project work
Wednesday	7.00am – 4.00pm	Evening football match		
Thursday	Day Off	Leisure centre am	Jobs at home Evening shopping trip	
Friday	Day Off		Clean car Gardening	10am – 12pm Morning study Project work
Saturday	1.30pm – 9.30pm	Swimming with sons am		
Sunday	7.00am – 4.00pm		Evening with family	

Julie is 18, she is employed in a community hostel working towards her NVQ at level 3. She has a boyfriend and enjoys discos, horse-riding and local church activities.

	Work	Leisure	Home	Study
Monday	8.00am - 5.00pm			8pm – 10pm Evening study
Tuesday	8.00am – 5.00pm		Jobs at home Evening	
Wednesday	8.00am – 5.00pm	Church activities		
Thursday	8.00am – 5.00pm			8pm – 10pm Evening study
Friday	8.00am – 5.00pm	Evening disco		
Saturday	DAY OFF	Evening disco	Clean bedroom morning	Project work 2pm – 5pm
Sunday	DAY OFF	Horse-riding morning Church evening		

Figure A1.2   Sample diaries

Time management techniques

All these techniques can be useful in your working life and at home, but you do not have to try them all at once. Remember that if you take one step at a time you are more likely to be successful. From your analysis of your time log, identify the techniques you feel would be most effective in *your* life.

Set goals and targets

It is of vital importance to establish at the outset just what it is you are trying to achieve. Set down a date by which that goal must be reached and a reasoned estimate of the time it will take daily, weekly and so on to realize that achievement. Examples are undertaking a course of study or improving your golf handicap for a forthcoming competition.

An examination date or date for submission of an essay may constitute an absolute deadline and occupy a certain number of hours of study per week to ensure a pass. After study time, and taking into account duty and domestic calls, have you sufficient time left to put in the necessary practice on the golf course to realize that other objective?

Goals and targets must be realistic or you will wind up with a number of projects only partially completed.

Define priorities

In order to ensure that goals are reached, it is essential to set down on a daily, weekly and monthly basis a note of things which *must be done*, and things which *should be done if possible*. You would find it helpful to note down alongside each target an estimate of the time it will take to complete the task.

Use a diary

A most useful tool for the definition of priorities is a diary. Beware, however, of the dangers of the large desk diary which, because of its size, creates the temptation to enter too much detail, thereby wasting more time! A pocket diary is quite adequate for noting only your *must do* and *should do* headings, and by its size need never be far away from your hand. Do enter all your *must do* and *should do* tasks, including domestic and leisure commitments as well as those tasks relevant to business or study.

Prepare a plan

A study plan is merely a timetable in which you may well include a note of the *must do* items from your list of priorities.

Delegate

Study of your time log may well reveal that you are doing things which other people in the organization are perfectly capable of doing, or that you are meddling in activities which colleagues or subordinates are already executing well. Remember that people are flattered by being asked to undertake a task on your behalf, by your demonstrating your confidence in their ability to complete that task satisfactorily. As a result they will react in a positive way. Perhaps on the first occasion the task will take a little longer than if you did it yourself. The extra time taken, however, is unlikely to be critical. Additionally, you should always be available and prepared to answer questions on the task to be delegated. You will find that on subsequent occasions the questions become fewer and fewer as the relative, colleague, friend, subordinate or whoever becomes familiar with the routine involved.

Communication

Communication is important. In planning your week remember that other people can help you with your plans, but they do need to know what it is you want done, when it must be completed and how and when they can help. Good communication, too, is an essential part of the art of delegation.

Review

Review your plans as you go along to check out where the time is going. Have you achieved your targets? Do you need to make any changes? Do you need to alter your priorities? Your plan as originally written will almost certainly be revised time and time again in the light of experience or in the wake of some mishap or unexpected event, or as a result of dramatic changes in your circumstances or expectations.

It may take you a while to become accustomed to managing your time in this way, but when you see the benefits you will realize how much more control you have in your life. In addition you will almost certainly feel more relaxed and fulfilled.

Some time-saving tips

As you will see, they cover "time" from a variety of angles. This is because time management is something that can affect all aspects of your life, if you want it to.

- Do your "thinking" on paper. You will make quicker and better decisions if you write down the pros and cons of a line of action. This does not use up time, it saves time!
- Make sure you get a reasonable amount of exercise every day. This not only promotes health but reduces fatigue to help you make the most of "prime time".
- Avoid clutter. Time is wasted in searching for what you want. For example, plan each night what books, notes, equipment you are going to need next day, and lay it out ahead of time. Do *not* do this for other members of the family – delegate that task!

(ii)

Using the library

Gillian Senior

During your support worker course, you will undoubtedly be required to find information relating to your area of work and to seek help with any projects or assignments necessary to the course. In order to fulfil your informational needs, it is essential that you become familiar with using a library.

Libraries have in the past earned the unfortunate reputation of being rather daunting and unfriendly places. This is no longer the case because they adopt a more user-friendly approach. By familiarizing yourself with your library, discovering its services and facilities, arrangement and procedures, you should become a confident and successful library user.

This appendix covers the following topics:

- Types of library
- Familiarization
- Arrangement of library stock: books, journals and other resources
- Undertaking a literature search
- Obtaining information

Types of library

Library facilities vary considerably from one area to another, so check what is available to enable you to make full use of the services and resources.

You may have access to a range of services within your Trust or college, from large multidisciplinary libraries catering for all levels of health care staff, to small units. Many will fall somewhere between the two.

Your health authority may also have other separate facilities, such as Health Promotion Units dealing with health education issues, or information departments which are concerned with the collection of local health statistics.

Public libraries can provide a wealth of general information which may be useful to you and these too should be explored and used.

You may also be allowed to use your local college or university library facilities, but these are usually for reference only and it is unlikely that you would be able to borrow books. Individual organizations often have their own specialist libraries and information centres. They are usually able to send out information in the form of leaflets and booklets, if you contact them.

Check with your assessor, who should be able to advise you of the libraries to which you have access.

Familiarization

When you have discovered which library or libraries may be most appropriate to your requirements, it is essential that you learn how to use them effectively.

A visit to your local medical/nursing library may be incorporated into your training programme. If not, contact the librarian and ask to be shown around. If you do wish to visit, it might be worth while organizing a small group visit rather than everyone visiting independently.

When you arrange a visit, you will need to find a variety of general information which will be unique to each library. There may already be a printed guide listing the services and facilities available. If not then make a note of some of the basic information you will require, such as:

- opening hours
- staff availability (in some smaller health libraries, this may be different from the opening hours)
- range of stock (subjects available, books/journals etc.)
- borrowing arrangements (how many/ for how long/can they be renewed/are there fines for overdue books?)
- photocopying facilities
- how to use the catalogue
- type of classification scheme (i.e. arrangement of books)
- interlibrary loan facilities.

It is usually the range of stock that is the determining factor when you decide which library will be most useful to you. However, collecting the above information may help you to organize yourself more effectively – for example by knowing if a library is open in the evening or at the weekend.

Remember that the library staff are there to help you. Do not be afraid to ask them for assistance.

Books

The collection of books in the library will be arranged by a **classification scheme**. There are a number of these schemes: for example, public libraries often use the Dewey Decimal Classification scheme (DDC), which is also popular in medical/nursing libraries, along with the National Library of Medicine scheme.

The reason for using a classification scheme is to allow books on the same subject to be shelved together, with related subjects close by. This allows you to browse easily through books on similar subjects.

Most libraries will have a list of subject headings available, to enable you to look up your topic, find a relevant classification number and locate the book on the shelves. Reference books may be kept in a sequence separate from those which are available for loan.

Catalogues

The library will have a record, or **catalogue**, of the books which it holds in stock, and possibly those to which it has access in other libraries. The catalogue may be available in a number of formats: as cards, as microfiche, or (increasingly common) as computerized data.

You will need to learn how to use the catalogue, in order to check for the books which are available on topics of interest to you. Your library may have a guide to show you how to use the catalogue, but if not, ask a member of staff to show you. If you are not using the catalogue properly, you may miss relevant information.

Whatever the form of the catalogue, each "entry" should give you at least the following information:

author, title, place of publication, publisher, date of publication, classification number, and number of copies available.

A catalogue is useful to show the range of books available on a particular topic. This

is not usually possible by simply checking the shelves for books, as many may already be on loan.

Bibliographies

These are lists of references to books and related materials, usually arranged by subject. They do not relate directly to the stock held in your library, but will give an indication of what is generally available on a particular topic. Examples are *British National Bibliography* and *British Books in Print*.

Journals

Journals will be arranged separately from the book stock. Current issues are often kept on display, with back issues arranged in alphabetical order by title and then bound or boxed in chronological (date) order.

In order to trace information on your topic in the journals, you will need to find out what bibliographic tools are available. These come in a variety of formats.

Indexes

These are lists of references to journal articles, usually arranged by subject. Examples are *RCN Bibliography*, *AJN International Nursing Index* and *Index Medicus*.

Abstracts

These are lists of references to journal articles and books, together with an abstract (summary) of the content. Again they are usually arranged by subject. Examples are *DHSS Nursing Research Abstracts* and *ASSIA Applied Social Sciences Index and Abstracts*.

Computer databases

Many medical/nursing libraries now have computerized facilities for undertaking literature searches for journal articles. One popular system is known as a CD-ROM (compact disc read-only memory). These databases are updated regularly and contain a wealth of information from international nursing and medical journals.

Examples are *CINAHL Database* (for nursing literature) and *MEDLINE Database* (for medical literature).

You will need to read the instructions to any index or abstract you check, to understand how it is arranged, and check the range of subjects it covers.

Other information

Libraries do not deal simply with books and journal articles but may have other collections of information which could be of interest to you. Examples are audio-visual resources, newspaper cuttings, leaflets and statistical data. Make time to explore the libraries you use to discover what other resources are available. There may be separate catalogues or lists of these collections, so check with library staff.

Undertaking a literature search

When you have considered the libraries to which you have access and decided upon the ones which are most appropriate to your requirements, you will need to start looking for information. Allow yourself plenty of time to search – it often takes much longer than you anticipate. Remember that libraries are busy places and you may have to wait to speak to staff or to use the computer database, computerized catalogue or photocopier.

Consider which of the bibliographic tools (discussed in the section on journals) you are going to use. You may need to check a number of these in order to obtain the information you require. Library staff will be able to advise you on which are the most appropriate.

Write down your topic area and try to think of any other subjects which may be related to it. You may also need to think about the terminology you are using, noting key words and alternative headings which may be appropriate. Use dictionaries and encyclopaedias to find these. If you check an information source and are unable to find a subject under the heading of your choice, then use one of the alternatives instead.

If you are looking, for example, at "Patient discharge planning", then different information sources may list it under different headings:

- *RCN Bibliography* lists it under "Continuity of care"
- *AJN International Nursing Index* lists it under "Patient discharge"
- *The CINAHL Database* lists it under a variety of terms: "Patient discharge", "Continuity of patient care", "Discharge planning".

You should also be aware of American terminology if the databases of indexes you are using are of US origin. Information may be listed under headings which are not immediately obvious to you. For example, pressure sores may be listed under "Decubitus ulcers".

Do not be overambitious when gathering information. You may have to consider the time-scale you have to complete your assignment and refine your search accordingly. You could limit your literature searching in a number of ways:

- by date (e.g. look only at information published after a certain date)
- by place of origin (e.g. look only at British research, rather than American or international)
- by types of information (e.g. are you going to include statistical data, audio-visual materials?).

Make sure you keep a record of the references you find. This enables you to trace the item, and ensures you are able to quote the full reference in written work.

Referencing

There are a number of different methods of referencing books and articles. One of these is the Harvard system, in which you will need to keep a record as follows:

For a book
author(s) surname plus initials

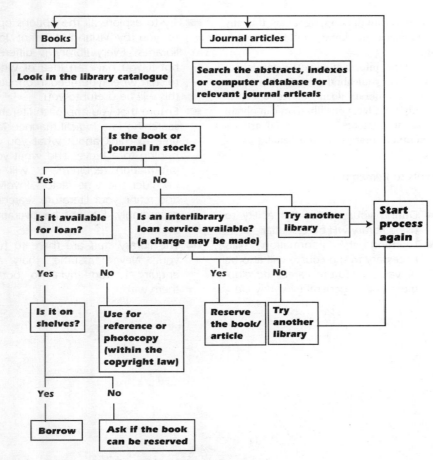

Figure A1.3 Finding books and journal articles

year of publication
title of book and edition
place of publication and name of publisher.

Example:
Luker, K. and Orr, J. (1992). *Health Visiting: Towards Community Health Nursing*, 2nd edn. (Oxford: Blackwell).

For a journal article
author(s) surname plus initials
year of publication
title of article and name of journal
volume number and part number
date and page numbers.

Example:
Fairlie, A. (1992). "Nurse–patient communication barriers", *Senior Nurse*, vol.12, no.3, pp.40–43.

Check with your assessor, who will advise you of the referencing system acceptable to your particular course.

Obtaining information

If the books you require are available in the library, you will probably be able to borrow them. However, you may be asked to complete a registration form first, and provide some proof of identity. If books are already on loan, you should be able to reserve copies, and will be notified when they are available.

Journals are often kept for reference only, although some libraries may let you borrow back issues. It might be more practical to photocopy the information you require, but you should ensure that you are within the Copyright Law. If in any doubt check with library staff before copying.

If the information you want is not available in your library, you could enquire if an interlibrary loan service operates. Usually for a fee, your librarian can obtain books or photocopies of journal articles from other libraries on your behalf.

Points to Remember

■ During your studies the ability to use a library will be essential.
■ Learning the information skills necessary to the course will also be of value in future career development and in general everyday life.

■ Try to explore all the options open to you by visiting different local libraries. Every library is different, but if you have an idea of where to start when you need information this will be useful to you.
■ Ensure that you approach literature searching in a logical manner. Take time to think about what you are hoping to achieve, and what your information requirements will be. Consider the time factors involved and refine your literature searching accordingly. Do not be overambitious.
■ The library staff are there to help you. Never assume that any enquiry is too trivial to bother them with.

In the current climate of employment where jobs are not plentiful and there is increasing competition for work, a prospective employee is more likely to secure employment if he or she is able to provide evidence of current competence. With the introduction of equal opportunities there is less emphasis on qualifications attained at school or college and more on the ability to function effectively at work.

Many people are realizing a need to compile a **personal portfolio**. There are several types in current use. The format you choose will depend upon the reason and purpose for which it is intended. It may take the form of a learning profile or could be a collection of evidence of what you can do.

With ever more mature people returning to education, new approaches to learning, more suited to the needs of adults, have evolved. Open and distance learning puts the responsibility for managing the learning process on to the student. This makes the development of a learning profile essential as the student needs to identify what they have to learn and how and where the learning will take place. It also enables the student to track their learning and helps with time management. The portfolio provides evidence of the person's ability to look objectively at what they can and cannot do.

The purpose of this book is to enable people to achieve an NVQ in care. If you have chosen to learn through a distance learning course, such as that offered by the Open College, the package will include help in developing a learning portfolio. Whether or not you are following a distance learning or other formal course, you will need to collect evidence of your competence in the workplace against which to be assessed. Putting this evidence together will be your proof of current competence.

What do you have already as proof of what you can do? For example you might have a driving licence or cycling proficiency badge. Have you done anything in the past, such as a first-aid course, where you collected evidence? Do you take photographs and put them together with mementoes of events special to you?

Collecting evidence

In practical work, as in caring, it may at first seem difficult to provide evidence of how well you do it. Look down this list of types of evidence and think what you have, or need, to demonstrate your competence:

- Being observed at work
- Products of your work
- Projects and care studies
- Questioning
- Explanations
- Testimonials
- Prior achievements

Observation of work practice

Being observed at work will form the basis for the greater part of your assessment. It is fairly straightforward for your assessor to sign your assessment record book to say you are competent at practical repetitive tasks; for example, testing urine. But how you interact with clients needs a written statement to confirm how well you do this. Your assessor may write notes on what you have done, but you may well be working alongside other professionals and their observations of your practice are equally important. Ask them to give you written comments on their observations of your work. This provides supporting evidence which can be included in your portfolio.

Example 1

"Mary has used her skill in giving information to a client, in a situation of a road traffic accident where the client was most anxious as to the whereabouts of his car. Mary liaised with the nurse in charge and was given permission to contact the local police station. The police gave Mary the necessary details which she immediately relayed to the client. Mary was conscientious in gathering the information by recording the names and location of the people she had spoken to. Her manner at all times was polite and appropriate to the level of understanding of the client. She was proficient in reporting all the

(iii)

Developing a portfolio

Kathleen Wheatley

relevant details to the nurse in charge."
S. Morris, Staff Nurse, 14 July 1995

Example 2

"Michael has participated fully in group therapies and has demonstrated his capacity to adapt to a different environment. He has shown initiative and sensitivity in dealing with a potential situation."   L. Jones, Occupational Therapist, 18 August 1995

Do make sure that any evidence you collect is dated and *signed* and, in the case of statements and testimonies, that the person writing the statement writes their name, job title and place of work. This may be needed for future reference.

Products of your work

Think what you do in your work which produces a written end-product. In a hospital or nursing home you may be given the responsibility of ensuring that certain clients drink sufficient fluids and pass urine. You will write this on a chart with name, date, times and signature. At the end of a 24-hour period you may add up the columns and calculate the difference between fluid taken and urine output. Photocopy this chart (*remember to remove the client's name to maintain confidentiality*) and keep it in your portfolio.

Alternatives to direct care observations would be taking telephone messages, recording stock balances and making appointments.

Projects and care studies

You may be doing a project or care study as part of course work. If it is small then the full written text could be put into your portfolio providing evidence of knowledge and understanding of a particular aspect of care. If the work is more than 1000 words it would be better to make a copy of the objectives, summary and the grading from your assessor. This would be sufficient evidence for portfolio purposes, bearing in mind that a prospective employer would not have the time at interview to read the whole work.

Questioning

Clients may ask questions about the service or care available. On occasions your assessor will ask about a range of aspects related to your work. Make a note of these questions and the answers you gave which demonstrated your knowledge and understanding.

Explanations

Carrying out a task demonstrates that you can *do* something. Being a competent carer also requires understanding. At the end of the day think about the tasks you have carried out and write an explanation of what you did and why you did things in that particular way.

Example 3

"I collected a urine specimen from Tom Brown's urinary drainage system. First I explained what I was going to do and why the specimen was needed so Tom would not be anxious and think there was something wrong. Then I collected a syringe and needle, specimen bottle which I labelled using a ballpoint pen – ink or fibre pens may blotch if the label gets wet. I labelled it, first checking the name and number with the case notes for safety. It's best to label the bottle before putting the urine in as I have to put on gloves to collect the specimen. Next I took the things I needed to where Tom was sitting by his bed and pulled the curtains so he would not be embarrassed. I put on my rubber gloves – this is to prevent contact with body fluid, in this case urine, as the HIV is found in body fluids and no-one can be sure who is not HIV-positive unless tests have been carried out."

This explanation provides evidence of knowledge and understanding and attitudes.

Testimonials

A testimonial can be a formal written commendation from someone for whom you have carried out work, or it may be a simple card or letter of appreciation from a client or colleague. These provide useful evidence to demonstrate endeavour or empathy.

Example 4
"Dear Ann,

I cannot tell you how much it meant when you stayed with me throughout my embarrassing investigations. The previous time I had been left alone and I was really frightened, but with you there holding my hand this time it was not bad at all. I shall never be frightened again.

Best wishes
Susan"

Prior achievements
Certificates you have achieved previously, whether or not directly related to your current role, should be included.

Any achievement is of value. Some provide evidence of ability to study, others may demonstrate leadership skills or the ability to function within a team. There may be elements for which you can achieve credit without further assessment, alternatively they may be useful as evidence for future employers.

Compiling your portfolio
Remember, this is *your* portfolio. There is no right or wrong way to put it together.

However, there are a few points to bear in mind.

When asked to show evidence, you need to be able to locate it quickly. Keep the system simple and clear. Begin with a personal profile and include:

- Name
- Qualifications, with names of awarding bodies and dates
- A resumé of your working life, interests and hobbies, your hopes and aspirations
- Have sections with titles such as "Assessment plans", "Assessment records", "Work experience" and "Courses attended".
- Use dividers and colour code, number or letter each piece within the section.
- Have a ring binder with space for additional items which can be put in throughout your career
- Remove sections as they become obsolete
- Update it regularly.

Conclusion
A personal portfolio is a means of presenting *evidence* of what you can do. It is an important part of your proof of competence and can be used for assessment, when seeking employment or further education. It could be the most important document you ever compile.

APPENDICES
Projects and presentation

2

(i)

Project development

Kathleen Wheatley

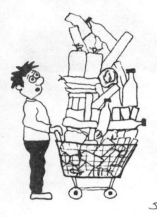

Project work is included in many caring courses, as part of the assessment process. This can be a daunting prospect. Once it is started, however, most people find that they really enjoy the work and get great satisfaction from the exercise. Starting is the most difficult part and a good plan of action will make the task much easier. Without a plan it is easy to become side-tracked and collect information from too many sources which then leads to confusion, wasted time, and difficulty in selecting the useful information. It is rather like going to a large unfamiliar supermarket without a shopping list – you collect a trolley-full of items you had not intended to buy and forget the items most needed, having spent too much money in the process.

Preparation, then, is the key to success. Plan a scheme of action and stick to it. Figure A2.1 summarizes the processes involved in project work.

The planning stage

Selecting the topic

The topic may be assigned to you, or choosing a suitable subject could be part of your personal development. If the decision is yours, then list several issues you would like to learn about or explore. Think these through in relation to the guidelines you have been given.

■ List the guidelines
■ Has the number of words you are allowed been stated?
■ Has the work to be based on the care of a single client or a group of clients?

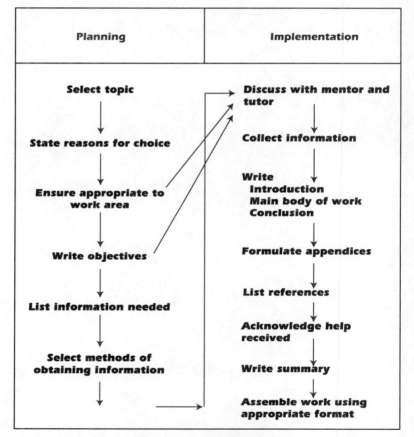

Figure A2.1   Planning and implementing project work

- Is it related to an Act of Parliament or a specific local issue?
- Decide which of the topics you have listed fulfil the guidelines or criteria you have to achieve.

The size of the project is important. Can you realistically undertake the topic in the time or number of words allowed? For instance, if you have decided to do "Infection control" this is a vast subject; it would be necessary to identify one area (for example handwashing) and research this in detail rather than to cover all aspects of infection control.

Why this topic?

Project work is assigned to enhance the learning experience of each student by allowing the student to take control of their learning. To get the most out of this experience it is important to be totally objective about the subject. Check your own objectivity by listing your reasons for the choice of subject. If there is an emotional or personal reason on your list, it is possible you have made the choice from a personal viewpoint. It could prove difficult not to let your own opinions and attitudes influence your work. If, however, your list includes words like "learn", "understand", "compare" and "contrast", then your choice is likely to be a good one.

Relationship to work

If the project work is directly related to the area in which you are working – community care, nursing home, hospital or child care – it will be much easier to collect data and enlist help from professionals within the care environment. Perhaps more importantly, it will be possible to use your new knowledge and understanding and may help or enable changes to improve the quality of care for your client group, or those caring for them.

Writing the objectives

It is essential to be clear about what you are going to do. This entails writing a list of what you are aiming to achieve – that is, the objectives.

Example

Topic: Reducing agitation in elderly clients
Objectives:
(a) To learn what causes agitation
(b) To identify the times of day/night when clients are most disturbed
(c) To compare different methods of reducing agitation.

You may feel that this is wasting time when you are eager to be getting on with the project, but listing objectives is crucial to the success of your work. It will save time in the end.

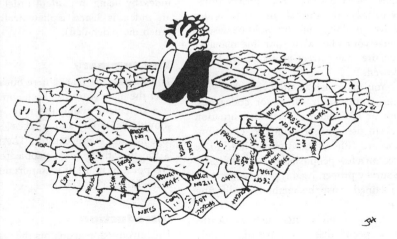

HAVING COMPLETED HIS PROJECT, JOE'S ONLY PROBLEM NOW WAS HOW TO GET OUT OF THE ROOM.

At this stage it is useful to have some confirmation that you are working along the right lines. Your mentor or assessor will be pleased to discuss the objectives with you. This will confirm that you are clear about your intentions.

Data collection

The objectives will give the clues to what data are needed to complete your work. Look at each one and decide what is needed in order to achieve it. Think about how and where you can find the information you will need to learn about the subject. This knowledge can be acquired from books, journals, and projects done previously by other students. Much of this information will be available in your library. Leaflets written for the public and health education packs can be obtained from the local health promotion unit.

There are organizations dealing with an infinite range of health and disease issues as well as charity associations and support groups, both local and national. Addresses for these are usually available in local libraries, health centres and health promotion centres. Having acquired the knowledge, the next stage is to apply that knowledge to your area of work. This may involve studying a client or a group of clients over a set period of time. For this, some form of checklist is required as a means of recording the observations. There may be ethical or legal issues involved in doing this. It would be wise to discuss your plan with your line manager to ensure that correct protocols are being followed.

You may wish to discover what your client group, their carers, or colleagues, think or feel about a particular situation or event using a questionnaire. Questionnaires are difficult to write and need to be tested on a few people before being used for the survey proper. Again, permission must be obtained to use this method of collecting data.

Statistics on events such as deaths from a specific disease are available locally and nationally. Some are published by government departments and local authorities. Your mentor or assessor will be able to help you locate the particular information you are seeking.

Project folder format

When all the information has been collected and the statistical data collated, the next step is to write up the work for presentation. There is a formal method for this which is easy to follow: Title page – Frontispiece – List of contents – Summary – Introduction – Main work – Conclusions – Appendices – References – Acknowledgements.

Title and frontispiece

The title page gives the first impression of content. It should capture the imagination and entice the potential reader to open the work and read on. A short title, written in large print, which informs the reader, is a good choice.

The frontispiece is the first page of the written work and should illustrate the title as well as listing the name and date of the course and the main aims of the work.

List of contents

The list of contents is placed at the beginning of the work. It should include page numbers and the main headings for each section. A list of contents differs from an index by being in content order (whereas an index is listed alphabetically and is much more detailed).

The summary

The summary is placed here but is written *after* the main work has been completed. It is a statement giving the main points. It should be brief and precise, bringing together the main features. The summary is the first thing most people read. With this point in mind, it is important to write it carefully.

Introduction

The introduction acquaints the reader with the subject he or she is about to experience. It should establish or initiate an interest in the work. It can be likened to the trailer of a

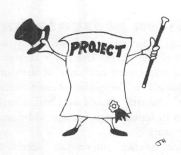

film, being a public relations exercise in promoting your work and persuading people that they really want to know the contents. It is important, then, that it is well-written. It is worth while testing the reaction of family or colleagues to your draft jottings.

The body of the project

The body is the main or central part which should be written in a systematic and logical manner, arranged in short chapters with a number of sub-headings. This will help to make the compilation easier and enable the reader/marker to identify how the project was undertaken, what methods were employed in collecting the information and how this was evaluated. *It must be stressed that clients, carers, institution, individuals or groups must not be identified by name or any other means, as this would breach the rule of confidentiality. Where a pseudonym has been used it must be made clear that this is the case.*

The conclusions

The conclusions are your beliefs or opinions based on reasoning, from the information and evidence you have gathered. This section may include how you have changed as an individual or as a carer. Under some circumstances it would be appropriate to make *recommendations*, but this must be done diplomatically and could be open to misunderstanding. As the con-clusions are the last part of the written work, they should leave a good impression. This can be achieved by ending with a positive statement.

The appendix

A number of pieces of information will have been collected which have not been used in the main work. These provide supplementary evidence to support the work. Leaflets produced by organizations or drug companies for patients' information, health promotion leaflets, graphs, charts, or diagrams, all come into this section. A blank copy of a questionnaire, if this method has been used, should also be included.

Each item should be numbered and referred to in the written work as "see appendix number . . . ". The appendix is a useful means of including a wide range of supporting evidence without copying.

This demonstrates the range of your research and enables the person reading or marking the work to check details not necessarily incorporated within the main text.

References

During your search for information you will have read sections from a range of books and other literature. You may have quoted sections from these. Any words, facts or numerical data must be referenced – that is, the source of information must be noted within the written work and a full reference written for each – see Appendix 1 (iii). Make a list as you use the information so that much time and effort can be saved in compiling this section.

Acknowledgements

Help and support, physical and emotional, will have come from a number of people. A list of names with expressions of thanks or gratitude acknowledges that you have appreciated their help and is a courteous gesture at the end of the work.

(ii)

Presentation skills

Kathleen Wheatley

A simple thing attractively presented creates a good impression by generating interest and anticipation of what is to follow. Marketing experts know this well and exploit the effects of psychological impact through advertising and packaging of their products. Using this technique for presentation of project work will produce the same effect. You are marketing your work to ensure that it is noticed and receives full credit. A little thought on how you can achieve this will be well worth while. Think of it as an investment, as supermarkets do when advertising one item greatly below its value in order to attract customers into the store. The way you package your work will enhance the contents.

Written presentation

The first point to consider is the visual impact of the cover. The cover creates a general impression not only of the contents but also of the quality of the contents within. The title should be short, clearly printed in letters large enough to be seen at a distance.

The overall impression needs to generate interest. This can be achieved by having a focal point. The focal point may be novel or very simple according to the subject. Vibrant colour cannot be ignored because very bright or strongly contrasting colours are eye-catching, but this has to be appropriate. For example, if the work was about death or bereavement a more sombre colouring with gold lettering would perhaps create the impression you desire.

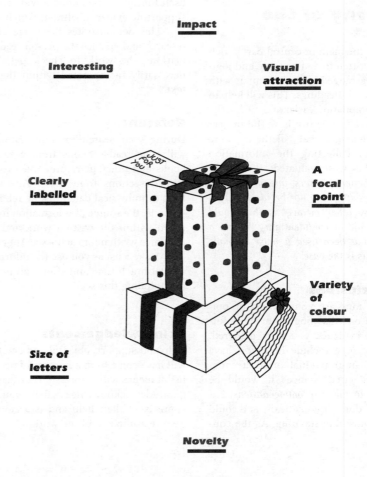

Impact

Interesting

Visual attraction

Clearly labelled

A focal point

Variety of colour

Size of letters

Novelty

Figure A2.2   Presentation skills

Quality of presentation

The quality of paper to be used and the folder or binding need consideration. All good writing materials tend to be expensive and this has to be borne in mind when deciding on the most suitable. If the writing is on one side only then it is possible to use a thin cheap paper. This type of paper tends to distort if adhesives are used to fix pictures or photographs within the text and would not be suitable for this purpose.

If the work is to be handled frequently then it is worth thinking about the use of a plastic cover to protect each sheet.

Work put into a folder without a binding is likely to become muddled unless it is clearly headed and colour-coded. There is also a tendency for sheets to be lost or removed. A binding of some nature is to be recommended. Ring binders are moderately priced and readily available. Additional pages can easily be inserted, so enabling the work to be updated. These tend to be the preferred method. Other methods to consider would be slide binders. These have the advantage of being cheap and do not require special equipment for fixing. The disadvantage is that they do not allow the pages to remain open without folding back the sheets.

Comb binders and heat binding give a more professional finish. Most colleges and offices have the facility to apply them. It is worth enquiring if you have access to such a facility.

Script

Typed work is uniform and neat. If you have access to a word processor this is by far the best method to use. As an alternative, many agencies will type work for you but this involves considerable cost. If neither method is appropriate then it is usually acceptable to present the project in the handwritten form. Your course guidelines should state if a particular method has to be employed.

Whichever method you choose, the rules to follow are:

- Use black ink.
- Head each section clearly.
- Use sub-headings within each section.
- Use double spacing throughout.

Diagrams

Each diagram should be labelled with what it represents. The use of colour may make the diagram easier to follow, particularly if it illustrates a sequence of events.

Numerical data

Numerical data are frequently illustrated through graphs and pie charts. These, too, should have a title heading, a brief explanation of where the data came from and what they represent. More information about presenting numerical data can be found in Appendix 2(iii).

Oral presentation

It is quite normal to feel anxious about giving an oral presentation. A little anxiety is useful as this causes adrenaline to be released and motivates the body and mind into action. However, too much anxiety could cause you to become flustered and lead to a muddled delivery. It is important, then, to get the balance right. If you are well-prepared you will still have "butterflies" on the day, but these will quickly settle down once you begin to concentrate on what you are saying.

Preparation

Preparation falls into two categories – preparation of what you are going to deliver and preparation of yourself. First consider the preparation of the content of your talk. Look at your work and pick out the salient points. Write these on *prompt cards* and number each card in sequence. Now prepare an introduction to your topic.

Try to avoid giving a lesson or lecture on the subject but rather say what you did and why you did it. If diagrams, numerical data or flow charts appear in your written work, these could be transferred on to *transparencies* for use with an overhead projector, or put on to *flip charts*. This will enhance your presentation by helping you to describe the sequence of events, and will also help your audience to understand what you are saying.

Practice your presentation and time yourself to ensure that you are not going to run over the time limit. Listen to yourself on a tape recorder. How do you sound? Is your voice loud enough? Will your voice carry to the back of the room?

Think about preparing yourself well in advance of the day. The clothes you wear will create an impact on your audience. Remember that you will be the focal point, so it is important to look good. Generally if you feel good then you stand tall and look confident. Choose clothes that you feel most comfortable in – they don't have to be new or special but should be clean and smart.

On the day you will feel nervous, but try to reduce the tension by practising some method of stress management such as breathing exercises. You may have learned these during your course, but if not, then you will find some helpful hints in leaflets produced by your local health promotion unit.

Speaking to your audience

Think about these questions: Which teachers do you enjoy listening to? How do they present formal lessons? Do you especially enjoy any particular TV presenters? If so, what is it that attracts you in their presentation? By thinking about these questions you can consider what sort of style would be the most effective and appropriate *for you*.

Giving a good presentation is a skill which anyone can achieve by learning to apply some simple techniques.

- Convey enthusiasm by being excited about your topic. If you are not, how can you expect your audience to be? Sound as if you are eager to tell them about it, even if you feel on this occa-

sion that you would rather be anywhere but where you are standing at the moment!

- Speak up: it is better to be too loud than to mumble. Try to avoid using too many "er's" and "um's". It is preferable to have a complete pause, because this allows time for your listeners to consider a point. A pause can also give you the opportunity to emphasize important points.

- Never read from a script. You may end up talking in a monotone and that by definition is very monotonous!

- Always avoid reading the OHP from the screen, because you will present your back to the audience. Using a separate copy avoids this. Do not try to put too much detail on the transparency and use lettering at least 6 mm high.

- Look at your audience as you would in normal conversation. Avoid transfixing your eyes on just one person or one point in the group, but look around the whole audience . . . and *smile*!

- Everyone has some mannerisms. Don't worry too much about yours unless you know that something you do is going to be particularly distracting – for example constantly throwing long hair over your shoulder.

- Finish your presentation on a positive note. The last thing you say will be the first thing people will remember.

- Invite questions from your audience and remain standing looking at them while you do so.

- Do not rush away as if you cannot wait to escape, but gather your visual aids together and walk away slowly, conveying confidence by your composure.

And *then* you can relax!

Caring for people in any setting requires the collection of a vast amount of detailed information. Some of this is in numerical form. Examples are a patient's blood pressure recordings, fluid balance, temperature and weight.

As well as using numbers in the workplace it is quite possible that you will be required to complete some form of project as part of your course. You may want to present numerical information visually in a clear and concise way. This appendix aims to give you some ideas and guidance to improve your skills in this area by looking at some basic mathematical terms and tools, examining some simple and effective ways of presenting numerical data.

SI units

The Système International d'Unités (SI) is now the accepted international measurement system. It is the standard system which is used for almost all numerical measurements in science, including of course medicine.

The SI has seven basic units, which are:

metre – unit of length (e.g. measuring height)

litre – unit of volume (e.g. measuring urine or fluid balance)

kilogramme – unit of mass (e.g. a client's weight)

degree celsius – unit of temperature (e.g. a person's "normal" temperature is regarded as 37°C)

joule – unit of energy (e.g. a chocolate biscuit may contain 400 000 joules)

pascal – unit of pressure (e.g. a blood pressure reading of 16 kPa/10.7 kPa is the same as 120 mmHg/80 mmHg

mole – unit of the amount of a substance, used mostly in physical chemistry (e.g. 0.9% sodium chloride, a normal saline infusion, contains 150 millimoles each of sodium and chloride ions per litre).

You are most likely to come into con-

tact with the first four of these units. Although the SI unit for pressure is the pascal, it is usual for blood pressure to be measured in millimetres of mercury (mmHg) – it will be a long time before all of the sphygmomonometers can be replaced!

Prefixes are used to turn all the units into appropriate sizes. Four are in everyday use. These are (using "metre" just as an example):

kilo- (k): times 1000, as in *kilo*metre
centi- (c): one-hundredth, as in *centi*metre
milli- (m): one-thousandth, as in *milli*metre
micro- (μ): one-millionth, as in *micro*metre

The first three sound fine (kilometre, centimetre, millimetre), but micrometre sounds a bit odd. That is only because we tend not to use such a small measurement in our everyday lives; if you were a precision engineer it would be very useful. In theory any of the other units could be substituted here for "**metre**". In practice we use some of the prefixes more than others.

Try it with grammes. Milligramme and microgramme sound fine but centigramme sounds a bit odd. It would be one-hundredth of a gramme. Similarly with litre, but here the odd-sounding one is kilolitre (a thousand litres).

Decimals

The first thing to remember when using decimals is to keep all the decimal points in line. This will prevent you from getting confused with the values. The chart below illustrates this and also reminds you of the values represented. Always insert the zero before the decimal point if there is no whole number (e.g. 0.1234), because it is easy to miss the decimal point if you just put .1234. (Try picking up 1234 kilograms rather than 0.1234 kilograms).

0.5	represents one-half
0.25	represents one-quarter
0.1	represents one-tenth
0.01	repesents one-hundredth
0.001	represents one-thousandth
0.0001	represents one-ten-thousandth

Using and presenting numbers

David Tordoff

0.000 01   represents one-hundred-thousandth

0.000 001   represents one-millionth

Placing the decimal point in the wrong place could have disastrous results. Receiving a drug dose which is 1000 times larger than what was prescribed is unlikely to be good for your health!

Rounding

Particularly when you are using a calculator, you will find calculations result in numbers with several decimal places. Often this will not be of much help and may give a false sense of accuracy. If you do not need a very high level of accuracy, or if there is doubt about the accuracy of the information itself, then you can present the result with a minimum number of decimal places or as a whole number. This is done by rounding the figure up or down, so 12.34567 becomes 12.35 (with two decimal places) or 12 (as a whole number).

Notice how we first look to the figure to the *right* of our cut-off point (12.34567) – if this is 5 or above then we round *up* (so we arrived at 12.35). If the figure to the right of our cut-off point is below 5, as in 12.34267, then we simply remove the numbers to the right (so 12.34267 becomes 12.34).

Percentages

This is another area where we tend to get a bit rusty if we don't use the calculations very often. If we are working with percentages then we are basing our calculations on the fact that the whole (e.g. 40 patients) is represented by 100 per cent (100%). Half of that group of patients could be described as 20 patients or 50%; quarter of the group as 10 patients or 25%; three-quarters as 30 patients or 75%.

Example 1

What is 8 patients as a percentage of 40 patients?

$8 \times 100 \div 40 = 20\%$

or

$\frac{8}{40} \times 100 = 20\%$ (either way works)

Example 2

What is 90% of 40 patients?

$40 \div 100 \times 90 = 36$ patients

or

$\frac{90}{100} \times 40 = 36$ patients

Whilst you can do these calculations by hand, it is certainly quicker and easier to do them with a calculator. Check with your own calculator's instructions and you may find a short cut such as:

$8 \div 40$ [%] (use % key) = 20%

or

40×90 [%] (% key again) = 36

Percentages are very useful when we are comparing things or trying to give some sense of proportion. If 23 of our 40 patients are female, then what is the percentage of females in the group? Using our calculation we find:

$23 \times 100 \div 40 = 57.5\%$

or if we use a calculator:

$23 \div 40$ [%] = 57.5

However, we do need to be careful how we use percentages. If the numbers are very small it is possible to give a false sense of importance. For example, "50% of the patients in the side ward are over 99 years old". How many patients are we referring to? If it is a side ward with ten beds then it would be remarkable to have five patients over the age of 99. If it is a two-bedded side ward then one patient aged 100 years would not be quite so remarkable.

Presenting information using numbers

When you are using rows of numbers it is worth making life as easy as possible for yourself and your reader. Which of the examples below is the easier to add up?

634.76092	634.76092	635
94.83654	94.83654	95
2654.23651	2654.23641	2654
1.25735	1.25735	1

The key is to use only as many decimal places as is necessary or useful and to make sure you keep them in line. Note that in the example above using only whole numbers, we keep the hundreds, tens and units in line. This makes the numbers much easier to deal with.

It is usually easier to understand the information being given by numbers if there is some form of visual aid. This is where graphs and charts are useful. Remember, poor data are not improved by good presentation but good data can lose their impact through poor presentation.

There are a few points to follow when using graphs and charts:

- Always give the diagram a title. This should tell the reader what it is about.
- A sub-title may be useful to explain the diagram's content more fully.
- Label the axes where necessary.
- Indicate what values you are using along the axes.
- Don't try to put too much information in at once. It may be more effective to use two diagrams than one cluttered one.

x **and** y **axes**

The convention is that the horizontal base line of a graph or bar chart is the x axis and this displays the "independent" variable (the information that is set – in the example that follows it is the age ranges). The vertical side is the y axis and this displays the "dependent" variable (the information that changes for each group – in our example the numbers within each age banding). If you were to turn the bar chart on its side (having the bars running from left to right instead of bottom to top) then the x axis would become the vertical and the y axis the horizontal, maintaining their relationship to the information.

Bar charts

To describe, for example, the age range and spread of a group, various types of diagrams can be used. Firstly we need usable figures that will give the required information. The 40 patients used in our previous example attend an outpatient clinic on a regular basis. Their ages are given below in years:

Females
15 53 74 21 35 93 87 45 67 23 64
46 83 63 26 73 54 51 36 48 42 76
90 72 83 28

Males
64 84 64 72 7 52 28 37 45 62 71
58 43 34

Putting the ages in ten-year groupings will be sufficient to illustrate the spread in this case. This gives the following breakdown:

0–9 yrs 0f/1m	10–19 yrs 1f/0m
20–29 yrs 4f/1m	30–39 yrs 2f/2m
40–49 yrs 4f/2m	50–59 yrs 3f/2m
60–69 yrs 3f/3m	70–79 yrs 4f/2m
80–89 yrs 3f/1m	90–99 yrs 2f/0m

We can now draw a bar chart to show the distribution (see Figure A2.3).

If we want to make the chart more informative we can produce separate bars for the males and females. This enables us to see at a glance any differences in age by gender for those attending the clinic (see Figure A2.4).

We can use slightly different presentations to show the same information. The principle remains the same. Note how the diagrams are labelled – we shouldn't leave anything for the reader to guess at.

Pie charts

Pie charts provide a useful way of displaying information but look complicated to construct. First think about what you want to display. A pie chart illustrates *relative amounts* and so is good for displaying percentages.

Now comes the problem – a circle has 360 degrees and most of us do not work with degrees very often!

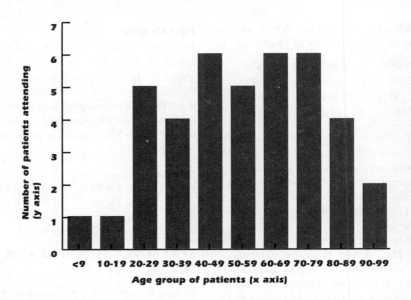

Figure A2.3   Outpatient attendances by age group

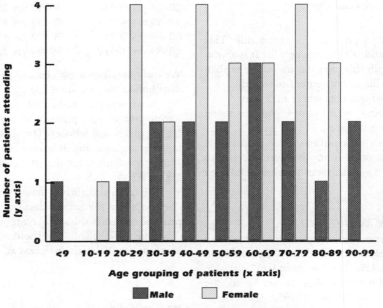

Figure A2.4   Outpatient attendances by age group and gender

Fortunately we can work with the fact that the whole circle is the same as 100%. Thus 1% = 3.6° (360° divided by 100). All we have to do is change the numbers into percentages and we can then work out how many degrees we need to mark off within the circle.

We can try this with the relative number of males and females within our sample. We have 14 men and 26 women. 40 = 100%, so 14 men make up 35% and 26 women 65%. (We can check our calculation by adding the two percentage figures. These should add up to 100%.)

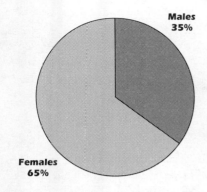

Figure A2.5 Outpatient attendances by gender

We know that 1% = 3.6°, so 35% × 3.6° = 126° and 65% × 3.6° = 234°. We can now construct our pie chart using a protractor to measure off the degrees (see Figure A2.5).

When using a pie chart do be careful not to put in too much information. It is very important that your reader can differentiate between the segments.

Using just bar charts and pie charts it is possible to display a wide variety of information effectively. You may, for example, want to show the comparative lengths of stay in hospital of a group of patients or their sources of admission. Bar charts would be ideal for this because they are especially useful for illustrating overall trends. If you wanted to demonstrate how the budget was allocated then using a pie chart would help to give a clear indication.

It is relatively easy to produce by hand the diagrams we have discussed although it can take a fair amount of time and effort. A simple way of producing a high standard of diagram is to use a computer. Many software packages can generate charts and graphs and it is well worth making enquiries to see if any are available to you (and if anyone is able to help you use them if you are not familiar with the package). You will still need the raw information and need to have a good idea of what you want to produce. The computer will simply do the easy bit – the drawing.

We have looked at presenting figures and data in isolation. Usually they are related to some text, for example a project. It is essential that a diagram or chart is never expected to "speak for itself". It should always be linked to the text. So, if you want to illustrate a point using some form of chart, refer to it in the text, particularly highlighting the major facts you want to emphasize.

Finally it is worth repeating that no matter how good the presentation, if the original information is poor it will be of little value. On the other hand, well-presented, accurate information will add a great deal to any presentation.

Index

Notes . . .

Notes